WHAT BIG PHARMA DOESN'T WANT YOU TO KNOW ABOUT ESSENTIAL OILS

Dr. Scott A. Johnson

Cover design: Scott A. Johnson
Cover copyright: Scott A. Johnson 2016

What Big Pharma doesn't want you to know about essential oils/Scott A. Johnson

ISBN-13: 978-0996413992

ISBN-10: 0996413995

Published by Scott A. Johnson Professional Writing Services, LLC

Printed by Create Space, an Amazon.com company

Discover more books by Scott A. Johnson at authorscott.com

allegedly arising from any information or suggestion in this book.

The Food and Drug Administration (FDA) has not evaluated the statements contained in this book. The information and materials are not meant to diagnose, prescribe, or treat any disease, condition, illness, or injury.

Contents

1

Big Pharma—The Modern-Day Goliath in the Health-Care Industry

The global pharmaceutical industry is nicknamed "Big Pharma" for a good reason. This enormous industry is a financial titan that has rapidly rocketed from about $400 billion a year in revenue in 2001 to a milestone of $1 trillion in 2014.[1] And this rapid pace is not predicted to slow anytime soon. Analysts anticipate that pharmaceutical industry revenue will eclipse $1.3 trillion by 2018. When you compare the nutritional supplement (nutraceutical) industry's revenue—which is expected to reach $175 billion by 2020[2]—it seems trivial. This battle for revenue and the dispute over what heath care should be between these two foes is a modern-day David versus Goliath. The only difference is the fact that Goliath is decisively winning presently. Like the Israelites in the Bible story of David versus Goliath,[3] the natural health industry appears dismayed and almost afraid to counter Big Pharma's attacks. But Big Pharma hasn't won just yet—brave David may be emerging from Saul's tent in the form of essential oils.

Big Pharma has lobbied and bullied its much smaller enemy, stifling its influence and making it more difficult to do business. Yet the savvy consumer—and one armed with evidence through this book—can cut through the rubbish and find natural options that replace the synthetic drugs pushed so heavily by Big Pharma.

Big Pharma's Unlimited Influence

Big Pharma's influence and power stretches to encompass prescribing physicians, medical education institutions, governments, regulatory bodies, policy makers, and consumers around the world. The United States, Japan, and China are the three largest pharmaceutical markets in the world. North and South America, Europe, and Japan account for 85 percent of the global pharmaceutical market. A staggering 1,367 paid lobbyists tirelessly pursue Big Pharma's interests and continued leverage over the US health-care system and, therefore, their grip on its population.[4] Big Pharma truly has built up a large head of steam that will take an impressive amount of force and courage to stop.

GLOBAL PHARMACEUTICAL MARKETS		
Country	Market Rank	Market Dollars
USA	1	$339,694,000,000
Japan	2	$94,025,000,000
China	3	$86,774,000,000
Germany	4	$45,828,000,000
France	5	$37,156,000,000
Brazil	6	$30,670,000,000
Italy	7	$27,930,000,000
UK	8	$24,513,000,000
Canada	9	$21,353,000,000
Spain	10	$20,741,000,000

Source: IMS World Review Analyst 2014

Given Big Pharma's overreaching influence on global lives, funding (could also be considered bribing) of key influencers, and intimidation of the public, they could be considered the twenty-first century's most powerful mafia. The industry reportedly spends over $3.2 billion annually lobbying US government officials to create and maintain policies favorable to Big Pharma,[5] this on top of the millions it spends on campaign contributions hoping to sway elected officials to see things the Big Pharma way.

In addition, Big Pharma currently spends one-third of all sales on drug marketing initiatives—more than double what they spend researching the safety and efficacy of these same drugs.[6] Savvy and persistent direct-to-consumer drug marketing has dramatically increased drug demand and produced an explosion of drug users in industrialized nations around the world. On the other hand, timely (spending more heavily at product launch) and incessant advertising to physicians has increased the dispensing of brands that spend the most marketing dollars.

Lastly, Big Pharma doles out millions of dollars to fund medical schools, which indoctrinates the next generation of doctors, firmly skewing their perception of medical care to join the drug-crazed frenzy. Even the professors of these schools aren't immune to Big Pharma's undue influence. Their research is largely funded by pharmaceutical companies, which can not only influence the outcome of the research but also have a lasting influence on the medical students involved. Big Pharma has pilfered and modified President Theodore Roosevelt's foreign policy of "speak softly, and carry a big stick" to "yell loudly, and maintain complete control of the big stick."

In other words, this colossal giant has massive influence over doctors, consumers, and governments to play the consummate bully and twist the global population's proverbial arm to get what it wants, when it wants it. The devastating consequence of Big Pharma's excess influence has created a population dependent on drugs to feel better.

Drug Use Doesn't Equate to Better Health
It is estimated that 70 percent of Americans currently take prescription drugs, yet Americans have the worst health outcomes of all industrialized nations. Of eleven countries analyzed in one recent study, the United States ranked dead last in health-care system performance, which measures the quality (safe, effective coordinated, patient-centered), access (cost and timeliness), efficiency, equity, health expenditures, and healthy lives in each country.[7] This despite the fact that the United States spends more for pharmaceuticals than the next top six counties spend on pharmaceuticals combined.

One of the major problems with direct-to-consumer drug marketing is the fact that these advertisements may drown out high-priority public health messages that encourage lifestyle behaviors (physical activity, proper nutrition, etc.) to improve health and prevent disease. These misleading advertisements are meant to persuade—not educate or inform—consumers that they have a need for a particular drug, and they often obscure messages regarding activity and nutrition that are the foundations of health.

Ill health is not caused by the lack of a drug; it is more typically caused by the consequences of poor eating habits and lack of physical activity combined with environmental factors. Unfortunately, our society has become a pill-for-every-ill society that not only seeks but also demands a quick fix for problems that have slowly occurred over months or years. Humans insist on being rescued from their poor choices without maintaining any accountability or demonstrating the willingness to change the habits that got them to the point of ill health in the first place.

In reality, Big Pharma advertisements may indirectly cause ill health by creating or exacerbating anxiety and stress surrounding normal experiences or symptoms. For example, you may have had a spicy fried meal that has left your digestive system in distress. You feel the classic symptoms of heartburn and indigestion and decide to watch television while you wait for it to pass. Of course, the advertisement playing during your show happens to be for a drug that treats gastroesophageal reflux disease (GERD). By the time the commercial is over, you are convinced it wasn't just the meal causing your symptoms, but that you have a medical condition that requires a drug. Your stress and anxiety rises as you consider the disease you now have, which releases hormones and chemicals that reduce digestive function, further exacerbating your condition. Armed with the persuasive information from the commercial, you march to your doctor's office practically baiting her to prescribe the drug you saw in the commercial.

Big Pharma's influence and power is bigger than ever before in recorded history, and the global population is paying the price—sometimes with their lives. Fierce greed is pervasive in Big Pharma as executives seek enormous profits over the health and well-being of the populations they serve. Executives drastically raise prices on medications used to prevent and treat life-threatening illnesses for the sake of padding their pockets. And the side effects and dangers of some medications are so high (often hidden by unethical safety studies) that the world is being poisoned slowly by synthetic chemicals foreign to the body.

Profits Over People

The business practices of Big Pharma suggest that they put profits far over people and their health. Here are just a few recent examples of how Big Pharma is about profits over people:

In 2015, Turing Pharmaceuticals purchased Impact Laboratories, including its drug Daraprim (a drug used to treat parasitic infections in those with a suppressed immune system). The contractual obligations that Impact Laboratories agreed to during negotiations effectively gave Turing Pharmaceuticals a monopoly on the drug, and in October 2015, they increased the price of Daraprim from $13.50–$17.50 per pill to $750 per pill—an unconscionable 4,000–5,000 percent increase. Was this a result of increasing drug development costs, a raw materials shortage, or excess demand? No—this was all about avarice and indifference to suffering.

Valeant was a company formed to be a drug-distribution company, rather than a full-fledged pharmaceutical company with research and development teams. The company CEO bought up competing businesses and fired their R&D teams—which he considered unprofitable—to acquire profitable drugs for distribution without having to invest millions into drug development. When Valeant acquired the drugs Nitropress and Isuprel (both drugs used to treat congestive heart failure), it tripled the cost of Nitropress to $805.61 per vial and increased Isuprel more than five-fold to $1,346 per vial. No explanation or reasoning was offered by the company's CEO for their drastic price increases, despite requests from the US Congress to justify the increases. This tactic was repeated with multiple other drugs that Valeant acquired, which suggests the company was simply seeking to pad profits.

For years, Big Pharma has produced nonsteroidal anti-inflammatory drugs (NSAIDs) to reduce the pain of millions of people. However, it didn't take long to discover that NSAIDs—particularly COX-2 inhibitors—increase the risk of heart attack and stroke. This was believed to be from long-term use, but more recent evidence prompted the US Food and Drug Administration to strengthen warnings for NSAIDs (both prescription and over-the-counter), emphasizing that heart attack and stroke risk increases even with short-term use. The FDA now admits that this risk can increase during the first weeks of NSAID use, regardless whether the person has or does not have heart disease.[8]

Acetaminophen is a common pain reliever and fever reducer, and Americans purchase products that contain it by the billions every year. But it is very likely that few who take it fully understand the risks they are assuming when they do. This drug accounts for more than one hundred thousand calls to poison control centers, and about sixty thousand emergency room visits each year in the United States. Acetaminophen is strongly associated with liver damage, and it is the leading cause of acute liver failure in the United States and other Western countries.[9] Regrettably, some of these cases of liver damage caused by acetaminophen have led to fatalities.

Considered one of the most dangerous drugs on the market, Actos (pioglitazone) was FDA approved in 1999 to treat type 2 diabetes. However, in 2007 use of the drug was associated with heart failure and a black box warning was added to the label to warn consumers of this risk.[10] Additional dangerous effects were disclosed when a long-term study by the drug's manufacturer, Takeda Pharmaceuticals, concluded that long-term use of Actos increased the risk of bladder cancer by 40 percent.[11] Based on these dangers, Actos was banned in Germany and France in 2011. But as of this writing, the FDA has chosen to ignore the hazards of this drug, instead choosing simply to add another warning regarding bladder cancer risk to the label.

Approved by the FDA in 2006, Gardasil (Gardasil, Silgard) is the human papillomavirus (HPV) vaccine created by Big Pharma to prevent cervical cancer. More recently it has also been recommended for boys to prevent HPV-related cancers of mouth, throat, penis, and anus. While vaccinations in general are controversial and extremely divisive, the HPV vaccine has been particularly scandalous.

The manufacturer of the vaccine, Merck, has been heavily criticized for its extremely aggressive marketing practices and lobbying campaigns to promote Gardasil as a mandatory vaccine.[12] Their fear-mongering marketing campaigns have created a panic among some parents who fear their daughter will die of cancer if they don't have the vaccine. This hardline marketing has led doctors to strongly and persuasively recommend the vaccine to unknowing adolescent girls and their parents at an average of $120 per dose and a recommended 3-dose course.

What Big Pharma is not telling you is that the vaccine is associated with thousands of adverse reactions, and regrettably some girls have died after receiving the vaccine. The CDC and FDA concluded that "Some deaths among people who received an HPV vaccine have been reported . . . [but] this does not mean that the vaccine caused the death, only that the death occurred after the person got the vaccine."[13] Nevertheless, 218 deaths following HPV vaccination are something to carefully consider before receiving this vaccine, particularly when so many of these deaths are occurring in children.[14] Side effects of the vaccine include: excessive fatigue, chronic headaches, nausea, stomachache, spontaneous abortion among pregnant women, widespread nerve pain, cognitive dysfunction, rapid heart rate, anaphylaxis, seizure, autoimmune disorders, disruption of the autonomic nervous system (the division of the nervous system that controls bodily functions not under conscious control), and a number of other serious side effects not currently reported in studies, but reported by recipients of the vaccine.[15,16,17,18,19] Gardasil appears to be another case of corporate greed and profits over people, with dire consequences to innocent children.

Creating Customers Not Cures

Sometimes one drug cascades into another drug, almost as if we are being set up by Big Pharma to require more drugs. A prime example is the stomach issues caused by NSAIDs. It is very common for those who take NSAIDs for any extended period of time to experience stomach discomfort and, in some cases, bleeding ulcers. What is Big Pharma's solution for this? It is to prescribe another drug—a proton pump inhibitor that blocks the production of an enzyme responsible for producing stomach acid. In turn, this leads to poor digestion, which may lead to subclinical deficiencies in nutrients, which eventually leads to ill health in another area. One only need to look at the lineup of medications required by many of our elderly parents to see that we are being lead down a path that requires the use of multiple medications.

Despite these blunders in the drug industry and the great risks to humans, the US Food and Drug Administration allows certain drugs to be fast-tracked through the FDA Fast Track Designation program. This program is intended to rush the development of and expedite potentially-dangerous drugs to market without undergoing the normal drug regulatory review process. The original intent of the program was to fast-track life-saving drugs desperately needed for public health, but this intent has been largely expanded to include other drugs now.

While the FDA claims this program is in the best interest of public health, experts suggest this process may pose serious safety problems. Indeed, a study of a similar Canadian fast-tracking process concluded that almost 35 percent of new drugs approved through an expedited process later received serious safety warnings or were removed from the market.[20] On the contrary, about 20 percent of drugs that go through the normal regulatory process are removed from the market or require serious safety warnings.

When you consider the elephant in the room of Big Pharma, you will usually fall on one side of the argument or the other. You will completely support pharmaceuticals as a testament to modern science and an advancement of the health of human kind; or you will hold disdain for the industry, its dangerous drug-peddling practices, and its death grip over health care in general. When you are considering whether to take a pharmaceutical or not, you must consider the risk-to-benefit ratio. Does the drug have a greater benefit than risk of harmful effects? In truth, all substances—even natural options—that have a positive effect can also have a negative side effect. What produces a positive benefit versus a side effect is the dose.

Although drugs do have their place in health care, greater preference should be given to the least invasive, but still effective remedy. If the benefits of a drug outweigh its risks, or if the drug is necessary to preserve life, a drug becomes a viable option. Conversely, if a natural option is available that will serve the same purpose as the drug, with less risk to the person, it should be the first option to consider. Applying this principle to human health and well-being puts people before profits, protects public health, and may reverse the unfavorable trend of throwing drugs at every problem facing today's man.

The best defense against Big Pharma's offense is education. This book is intended to arm you with a high level introduction to the deceptive practices of the pharmaceutical industry and reveal secrets that Big Pharma would rather remain concealed. What does Big Pharma want to keep hidden from the general public? What does Big Pharma not want you to know? They don't want you to know that new scientific discoveries are revealing that essential oils can replace many of the harmful medications being offered by Big Pharma with fewer side effects and a fraction of the cost.

2

Essential Oils—Natural Health's David

With the acceleration in the investigation and validation of natural remedies through science, one natural option has emerged as the frontrunner to contend with Big Pharma—essential oils. Essential oils unite the drug world of "rapidly effective" with the natural world of "reduced risk of adverse side effects." Aromatherapy, or better said, essential oil therapy, is one of the fastest growing therapies in the world today. These versatile molecules obtained from nature's most generous plants have the potential to improve a number of health conditions plaguing man, with far fewer risks.

What Are Essential Oils?

Essential oils are concentrated volatile extracts obtained from nature's most generous plants (seeds, bark, resins, nuts, rinds, leaves, grasses, flowers, twigs, and roots). They have been used throughout recorded history for spiritual, religious, ritual, food, cosmetic, and medicinal purposes. What makes them ideal remedies are their abilities to simultaneously act on the mental, emotional, spiritual, and physical aspects of well-being. When the body is in a more relaxed state—like that often achieved with essential oils—it is better able to carry out its normal healing processes. Once administered, these healing molecules travel throughout the body to the cells that need them most, to cleanse, repair, restore, balance, and revitalize.

Essential oils influence human health in three primary ways:

- Defend—Essential oils can protect the body against germs, toxins, harmful pathogens, and disease at the cellular level.
- Heal—Once in the body, essential oils travel to the tissues, cells, and organs that require them most, to heal, and restore balance, normal function, and homeostasis.
- Thrive—Essential oils work with the cells and support their vital functions, which leads to healthy tissues and organs, and ultimately organ systems and a body that thrives. This promotes the free flow of vitality throughout the body.

The Scientific Validation of Essential Oils

One needs only to search the term "essential oils" in the US National Library of Medicine National Institutes of Health to discover thousands of studies detailing the broad benefits to human health that they provide. Studies have confirmed that essential oils have antiviral, antibacterial, antispasmodic, anti-inflammatory, analgesic, antiseptic, antifungal, and antioxidant properties to name a few of what scientists have discovered.[21,22,23,24,25] And these are just the studies that have revealed benefits from essential oils obtained from a small number of known and commonly used plants. The number of essential oils from novel plants still waiting to be discovered on this vast earth is exciting to consider, especially when you contemplate what health benefits they may provide.

As science unravels the mysteries contained in essential oils, researchers have discovered that many essential oils have the potential to reverse disease and encourage health using the same pathways or mechanisms that drugs do. Indeed, science has revealed that essential oils can positively influence genetic expression to enhance overall well-being; influence the release of vital hormones and chemical messengers; enhance or restore normal organ functions: increase a person's ability to cope with stress; protect cells, DNA, tissues, and organs from damage; support a normal inflammatory response; and even slow or reverse aging.[26,27] A number of studies have even pitted essential oils directly against drugs, with the essential oils often demonstrating equal or better efficacy.

The Use of Essential Oils
Over the last two decades, essential oils have become more mainstream and popular. Hundreds of thousands of people have been introduced to the virtually unlimited potential of essential oils to influence human health and well-being. More of these individuals are discovering that regular use of essential oils as part of an aromatic lifestyle is both enjoyable and beneficial. This regular therapeutic practice of using essential oils promotes homeostasis and optimum well-being of the mind, emotions, body, and spirit. It is both an art and a science, and it offers rapid and far-reaching benefits for the human body when pure, authentic essential oils are used correctly.

Essential oils can be administered in four primary ways:

- *Inhalation.* The sense of smell is very powerful and connects us to our surroundings. Indeed, smell receptors are found throughout the body, suggesting that the sense of smell is vital to normal psychophysiological function.[28,29,30] Inhalation is a simple way to enjoy essential oils, but still offers profound benefits. This can be accomplished by simply inhaling directly from the bottle, adding a drop or two to a cotton ball or tissue, using an electronic diffuser, inhaling from an essential oil inhaler, or by adding a few drops to hot water.
- *Topical application.* Essential oils can be applied to the body, which allows them to enter the bloodstream without first being metabolized and altered in the digestive system. This is usually performed by diluting the essential oils in a carrier oil (such as almond oil, fractionated coconut oil, or grapeseed oil). Essential oils can be applied directly to the affected area, on the feet to stimulate reflex points, to the spine to influence the nervous system, to the chest or under the lip to also have an aromatic experience, or on many other places on the body.
- *Oral administration.* Some essential oils can be taken orally—preferably in a capsule. They can also be added to herbal teas, yogurt, honey, almond or rice milk, or other fatty substances. Adding essential oils to water is usually reserved for the mildest essential oils (like citrus essential oils). Another way to use essential oils orally is sublingually, or under the

tongue. This provides the essential oil direct access to the bloodstream through the rich supply of capillaries under the tongue. Again, mild oils should be used for this method.

- *Rectal or vaginal administration.* Some essential oils can be highly diluted and inserted through the rectum or vagina. This offers both localized and systemic benefits and bypasses much of the first phase of metabolism that occurs in the digestive tract. This method is often utilized among populations that have trouble swallowing or are experiencing nausea that may cause the essential oils to be lost if administered by mouth.

The Importance of Therapeutic-Grade or Medical-Grade Essential Oils

Unfortunately, because the essential oil industry has experienced tremendous growth, the quality of essential oils is becoming a greater concern. This explosion in the number of people who use essential oils regularly has placed some strain on the supply of pure, authentic essential oils. Demand for some essential oils is greater than some supplies, which leads unscrupulous suppliers to cut or adulterate their products with cheaper synthetic or natural compounds, or cheaper—but closely related—essential oils. In addition, this practice is sometimes used just to make more profit for those supplying essential oils to the industry.

Essential oils that consistently meet demanding standards established by the scientific community are most suited for professional and therapeutic use. These essential oils have gone through an array of tests to determine their quality, authenticity, and therapeutic value. They are free of synthetic compounds and produced according to the highest scientific standards.

Typical GC-MS of lavender (*Lavandula angustifolia*) essential oil.

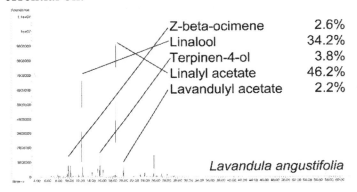

Z-beta-ocimene	2.6%
Linalool	34.2%
Terpinen-4-ol	3.8%
Linalyl acetate	46.2%
Lavandulyl acetate	2.2%

Lavandula angustifolia

Common Essential Oils Tests

Gas chromatography-mass spectrometry, or GC-MS for short, is a test used to separate the individual compounds in an essential oil and identify the relative percentage of each compound present. This test ensures that the appropriate compounds are present for the botanical species and may identify added compounds.

Optical rotation measures the direction and degree that polarized light rays rotate through a polarizer and then through the essential oil. If light rays don't rotate the direction and degree expected for a typical sample, it may identify adulterations or an inauthentic essential oil.

Refractive index measures the speed that light travels through an essential oil and compares it versus a standard. Adulterated and nontherapeutic essential oils will alter the speed of light.

Specific gravity measures the density of an essential oil against a known standard.

Organoleptic, or the human element, relies on the senses of a qualified expert to detect adulterated essential oils.

Microbial and heavy-metal testing ensures that the sample is free of pathogens, harmful organisms, and heavy metals.

Extracting Essential Oils

Extracting the highest quality essential oils requires strict attention to detail and a profound understanding of plants, distillation equipment, methods and time. The quality of essential oil obtained from the distillation process depends on a number of factors, including time, pressure, temperature, quality of distillation equipment, and quality of plant materials. Essential oils are extracted from plants by a number of methods, but the three most common methods today are steam distillation, hydrodistillation, and cold-pressing.

Steam distillation. The most common method used to extract essential oils, steam distillation introduces concentrated steam into a still that is full of plant materials. This process releases the volatile plant molecules, which are condensed back into a liquid and collected in a separator. The essential oils float to the top of the separator—on top of the water—and are removed by siphon. The water that is left over is another product called a hydrosol.

Hydrodistillation. Hydrodistillation (also called water distillation) is very similar to steam distillation, except that the plant materials are immersed in boiling water to extract the volatile molecules.

Cold-pressing. Cold-pressing or expressing is reserved for citrus oils, such as lemon, orange, grapefruit, and bergamot. A number of machines are employed to obtain essential oils from the rinds of these fruits.

Some essential oils, like ylang ylang, are distilled differently—called fractional distillation. During fractional distillation, essential oils are removed at different intervals during the distillation process. For example, the first essential oils may be removed one hour after distillation has begun, followed by a second fraction of essential oil removed between the second and third hours of distillation, and so on. Each fraction is considered a different grade of essential oil and contains varying essential oil compounds based on their volatility (the speed at which a substance changes from a liquid to a vapor, or solid to a vapor, and so on).

Very few essential oils are rectified. This practice involves the removal of unwanted or potentially harmful volatile compounds. For example, furocoumarins may be removed from bergamot to reduce the risk of photosensitivity, or minor sulfur compounds may be removed to improve the taste and smell of peppermint.

The Future of Essential Oils

The future of essential oils is bright as more and more science validates the traditional medicinal uses of these precious aromatic extracts. More people are seeking natural alternatives to harsh chemical drugs with potentially dangerous side effects, and essential oils are waiting to be discovered by these individuals. As more individuals discover the incalculable value of essential oils, they may truly become the David that the natural health industry needs. Then armed with a sling and a stone or two—or molecules and evidence—they teach Big Pharma that it can't play the bully any longer.

3

Transforming Your Medicine Cabinet

Prescription medications aren't the only thing that you need to worry about the risks of. Over-the-counter (OTC) medications don't require a prescription and are readily available at your local store, but that doesn't mean they are risk free. Refer back to the dangers of NSAIDS and acetaminophen—both of which are widely available without a prescription—to see what risks may be lurking in your medicine cabinet. Americans spend billions of dollars on OTC medications for everything from headache to indigestion. These medications can be taken safely, but they also pose risks, especially if they are used incorrectly or in combination with other medications. OTC medications pose a particular risk for children and infants who are more susceptible to their toxic and harmful effects. This all goes back to our risk versus benefits, and preference for the least invasive remedy that is still effective discussion. It is up to each individual to determine whether the benefits of drugs outweigh the risks.

If you prefer more natural options, essential oils make great replacements to synthetics when you want to support your health and well-being. What makes them ideal choices for your medicine cabinet? Here are several key advantages that they offer.

Multifaceted approach to wellness. As mentioned, they work simultaneously on the emotional, physical, mental, and spiritual levels of health. It is naïve to believe that ailments are purely mental or physical, spiritual or emotional. When you have a headache, it's not just the pounding pain in your head (body) you experience—you also experience an overall decrease in emotional and mental well-being. A remedy that can target multiple aspects of wellness at the same time is key to realizing greater wellness.

Long shelf-life. If you store essential oils unopened in a cool, dark place away from heat and sunlight, they can last a long time. In fact, some essential oils get better with age (sandalwood, patchouli, and vetiver to name a few).

Easy to use. Even responsible children are able to drop essential oils from a bottle to achieve results. It is so easy to inhale, apply, or take essential oils that it just takes some common sense and reasonable guidelines to make them work for you.

Potency. Essential oils are highly concentrated, which allows them to provide rapid correction, regeneration, and balance with few unintended side effects. They are so potent that often a drop or two is all it takes to get desirable results.

Safety. When used reasonably, and according to evidence-based guidelines like those found in *Evidence-Based Essential Oil Therapy*, essential oils are very safe. Users who follow practical and reasonable guidelines are less likely to experience any unintended results.

Versatility. Drug companies can only dream of a single drug that could potentially influence dozens to hundreds of health conditions. Yet that is what is found in essential oils. Because they are complex plant extracts with dozens to hundreds of molecules, they possess multiple therapeutic properties and myriad health benefits in one single essential oil.

According to the American College of Preventive Medicine, the most commonly used oral OTC medicines include those used for cough/cold, allergies, pain relief (analgesics), antacids, laxatives, and diarrhea.[31] The most common topical medicines are used for toothpaste, oral antiseptics and rinses, first aid treatments, lip remedies, and eye-care products. When it comes to children, by far the most common medications are analgesics and fever-reducers like acetaminophen and ibuprofen. Other commonly used OTC medications include those used for congestion, earache, sore throat, indigestion, constipation, and sleep.

The most common prescription medications depend on whether you determine this total by sales volume or number of prescriptions. But common prescription medications include hypothyroid medications, antidepressants, cholesterol-lowering drugs, proton pump inhibitors, asthma medications, high blood pressure medications, attention deficit drugs, diabetes medications, and antiepileptics.

Although essential oils can correct health conditions using similar pathways and with similar mechanisms of action as drugs do, it is very important that you include your medical professional in your health decisions. Always check a well-researched reference like *Evidence-Based Essential Oil Therapy* for any cautions with children, medications, and health conditions before using essential oils. It can be a wonderful experience to partner with a medical professional who is willing to consider your desires to use natural products and who has a basic understanding of evidence-based natural options. Preference should be given to the least invasive/risky option, and the benefit-to-risk ratio should be considered with your medical professional before making a decision.

Do not alter any medical treatment or the use of medications without the permission of your medical care provider. Consult your doctor or pharmacist before taking any essential oils with medications or for certain health conditions. Statements in this book have not been evaluated by the FDA. Information herein is not intended to be taken as medical advice. FDA regulations prohibit the use of therapeutic or medical claims in conjunction with the sale of any product not approved by the FDA.

4

Allergy Medications

Allergy medications—both prescription and OTC—are used to inhibit an improper immune response to substances (allergens) the body considers intruders. When an allergen enters the body through ingestion, inhalation, or contact with the skin or mucous membranes, white blood cells release an antibody that binds to mast cells. Mast cells rupture (degranulate), which releases immune chemicals like histamine that increase inflammation in an effort to combat the allergen. This overreaction by the immune system causes the classic symptoms of allergies—water eyes, runny nose, scratchy throat, sinus congestion, and rash.

Allergy medications come in various forms, including pills, liquids, shots, eye drops, inhalers, nasal sprays, and creams. Antihistamine allergy medications block cellular histamine receptors' response to histamine. Decongestants reduce the swelling of blood vessels in the nasal airway to make breathing easier. Corticosteroids suppress the immune system, which reduces inflammation. Another class of allergy medications is mast cell stabilizers, which work by blocking the release of immune system chemicals from mast cells that are involved in allergic reactions.

Side effects (depends on the class of allergy medication used)
- ✓ Drowsiness

✓ Dizziness
✓ Weakness
✓ Insomnia
✓ Constipation
✓ Upset stomach
✓ Dry mouth, nose, or throat
✓ Difficulty urinating
✓ Blurry vision
✓ Nosebleed
✓ Headache
✓ Nausea or vomiting
✓ Cough
✓ Fungal infections
✓ Stinging or burning sensation in the nose
✓ Cough
✓ Flu-like symptoms
✓ Bad taste in the mouth
✓ Discoloration or thinning of the skin

Essential oil alternatives

➢ Cedarwood (*Cedrus deodora*) essential oil balances mast cell degranulation, which may help reduce inflammation and allergies.[32]

➢ German chamomile (*Matricaria recutita*) essential oil blocks mast cell degranulation to reduce the severity of the immune response to allergens.[33]

➢ Lavender (*Lavandula angustifolia*) essential oil blocks mast cell degranulation when applied topically or injected.[34]

➢ Lemongrass (*Cymbopogon citratus* or *Cymbopogon flexuosus*) essential oil suppresses the release of the antibody IgE (an antibody involved in allergic responses), which subsequently prevents the release of immune chemicals by mast cells.[35]

➤ Tea tree (*Melaleuca alternifolia*) essential oil reduces histamine-caused allergic skin reactions.[36]

➤ Lemon (*Citrus limon*) essential oil has been used with other essential oils (niaouli and ravensara) in an inhaler to reduce allergic rhinopathy (nasal congestion, drainage, and obstruction of nasal passages).[37]

➤ 1,8-cineole, found in abundance in eucalyptus (*Eucalyptus globulus*) essential oil, reduces airway inflammation and the excess production of mucus.[38,39,40]

➤ Pine (*Pinus sylvestris*) enhances the production of airway surface liquid, which traps inhaled particles and influences the secretion of mucus.[41]

How to use the essential oils

Oral—Add 2 drops each of cedarwood, lavender, lemongrass, and German chamomile to a capsule and take up to 3 times daily.

Nasal Inhaler—Add 5 drops of balsam fir (*Abies balsamea*), 3 drops of myrtle (*Myrtus communis*), 3 drops of eucalyptus, and 3 drops of peppermint (*Mentha piperita*) essential oils to the cotton part of a nasal inhaler and use the inhaler every 15 minutes for 60 to 90 minutes, then every 2 hours as needed.

Steam Inhalation—Place 1 drop each of myrtle, eucalyptus, peppermint, and balsam fir in hot water and inhale for 10 minutes every 2 to 4 hours.

5

Antacids, Proton Pump Inhibitors, and H2 Blockers

Antacids relieve indigestion and heartburn by reducing the production of stomach acid. Antacids come in various forms including sodium bicarbonate, calcium carbonate, aluminum-based, magnesium, alginic acid, and aluminum-magnesium combination antacids. They are usually chewable tablets.

Proton pump inhibitors (PPIs) decrease the amount of acid produced by glands in the lining of the stomach. PPIs are used to treat acid reflux, peptic or stomach ulcer, and damage to the lower esophagus caused by acid reflux. These are often the first drug prescribed if an *H. pylori* (a type of bacteria that lives in the digestive tract and is strongly associated with stomach ulcers) infection is suspected as the cause of the ulcer. They are available as capsules or tablets and should be taken thirty minutes before the first meal of the day.

H2 blockers also target glands in the lining of the stomach to reduce stomach acid production. They thwart the action or histamine on parietal cells (cells in the stomach) that produce stomach acid. H2 blockers treat gastroesophageal reflux disease (GERD), or acid reflux. They are usually taken orally twice per day but may also be injected.

Side effects

Antacids

- ✓ Diarrhea (magnesium antacids)
- ✓ Constipation (calcium or aluminum antacids)
- ✓ Kidney stones (rarely, calcium antacids)
- ✓ Calcium loss and weak bones (aluminum antacids)
- ✓ Gallstones in children (calcium antacids)
- ✓ Renal insufficiency (calcium antacids)
- ✓ Metabolic acidosis (calcium antacids)
- ✓ Excess calcium in the blood (calcium antacids)
- ✓ Rebound acid reflux—increased acid production thirty to sixty minutes after antacid use
- ✓ Encephalopathy—kidney failure patients (aluminum antacids)
- ✓ Interference with drug metabolism and absorption

Proton Pump Inhibitors

- ✓ Headache
- ✓ Diarrhea
- ✓ Constipation
- ✓ Nausea
- ✓ Itching
- ✓ Bone fractures
- ✓ Infections (pneumonia, *C. difficile*)
- ✓ Drug interactions (clopidogrel—a drug used to prevent blood clots)
- ✓ Iron and B12 deficiency

H2 Blockers

- ✓ Constipation
- ✓ Diarrhea
- ✓ Dizziness

- ✓ Headache
- ✓ Hives
- ✓ Nausea or vomiting
- ✓ Difficulty urinating
- ✓ Abdominal, back, joint, or leg pain
- ✓ Blistering, burning, or redness of skin, hands, or feet
- ✓ Changes in or blurred vision
- ✓ Coughing
- ✓ Difficulty swallowing
- ✓ Difficulty breathing
- ✓ Slow heartbeat
- ✓ Flu-like symptoms
- ✓ Inflammation of blood vessels
- ✓ Mood changes
- ✓ Muscle cramps
- ✓ Unusual bleeding or bruising

Essential oil alternatives

- ➤ Ginger (*Zingiber officinale*) essential oil increases gastrointestinal motility (the speed that food travels through the digestive tract) as well as well as the GERD drug metoclopramide.[42] Decreased gastrointestinal motility is associated with GERD.[43] Ginger essential oil also inhibits *H. pylori* growth.[44]

- ➤ Myrtle (*Myrtus communis*) and spearmint (*Mentha spicata*) essential oils eliminates *H. pylori*, which may protect against stomach ulcers.[45,46]

- ➤ Cardamom (*Elettaria cardamomum*) extracts provide better protection against stomach ulcers than Zantac (ranitidine).[47]

> ➤ Clove (*Syzygium aromaticum*) essential oil stimulates the production of the mucosal lining of the stomach to protect against ulcers.[48]
> ➤ Copaiba (*Copaifera langsdorffii*) protects the stomach against ulcers caused by NSAID use.[49]
> ➤ Ethanolic extracts of marjoram (*Origanum majorana*) helps restore the mucosal lining of the stomach.[50]
> ➤ Oral administration of limonene, a compound abundant in citrus essential oils, helps relieve heartburn and GERD symptoms.[51,52]

How to use the essential oils

Oral—Take 5 drops each of lemon and ginger, and 2 drops of clove essential oil in a capsule up to 3 times daily, preferably with a meal (adults only).

6

Cholesterol-Lowering Drugs

If your cholesterol levels are high, your doctor may prescribe cholesterol medication to lower "bad" LDL cholesterol and triglycerides, and mildly elevate "good" HDL cholesterol. These drugs include statins, niacin, bile acid resins, fibric acid derivatives, and cholesterol-absorption limiters.

Statins are the most common drug prescribed and work by blocking the enzyme (HMG-CoA) responsible for the production of cholesterol in the liver. Statins may also help reabsorb existing cholesterol from the arteries.

Niacin is a B vitamin that mildly decreases LDL cholesterol and reduces triglycerides up to 30%, but it has a greater effect on increasing HDL cholesterol (up to 35%).[53] Unfortunately, synthetic niacin is often recommended by physicians, which is four times less absorbable than a whole-food source of niacin.[54]

Bile-acid resins (also called bile acid sequestrants) are substances that bind to bile in the intestines and prevent them from being reabsorbed. The body produces more bile to replenish lost stores. The liver requires cholesterol to produce bile, so it will take cholesterol from the blood, effectively reducing LDL cholesterol levels. Small doses may reduce LDL cholesterol by up to 20 percent.

Fibric acid derivatives, or fibrates, lower triglycerides and increase HDL cholesterol, but have very little effect on LDL cholesterol. They do so by activating a protein (PPAR-alpha) that stimulates the enzyme lipase, which ultimately decreases the production of triglycerides and increases HDL cholesterol.

Cholesterol absorption limiters (also called cholesterol absorption inhibitors) reduce the amount of cholesterol that your body absorbs by selectively preventing the absorption of dietary and biliary cholesterol. They are normally only prescribed to people who are unable to take statins.

Side effects
Statins
- ✓ Memory loss
- ✓ Mental confusion
- ✓ High blood sugar and type 2 diabetes
- ✓ Coenzyme Q10 (CoQ10) deficiency

Niacin
- ✓ Itching under the skin
- ✓ Flushing (warm, red, or tingly skin)
- ✓ Mild dizziness
- ✓ Sweating or chills
- ✓ Nausea
- ✓ Diarrhea
- ✓ Insomnia
- ✓ Leg cramps
- ✓ Muscle pain

Bile acid resins
- ✓ Heartburn
- ✓ Gallstones
- ✓ Bloating and excessive flatulence

✓ Constipation
✓ Abdominal pain
✓ Diarrhea
✓ Increased liver enzymes
✓ Cramping

Cholesterol-absorption limiters

✓ Breathing difficulty
✓ Swelling of the lips, face, tongue, or throat
✓ Hives
✓ Nausea
✓ Muscle pain, weakness, or damage
✓ Abdominal, back, or joint pain
✓ Skin rash
✓ Stomach upset
✓ Diarrhea
✓ Headache
✓ Fatigue
✓ Pancreatitis
✓ Hepatitis

Essential oil alternatives

➢ A combination of lavender (*Lavandula angustifolia*), basil (*Ocimum basilicum*), and monarda (*Monarda fistulosa*) essential oil has been shown to reduce cholesterol buildup in the aorta.[55]

➢ Cinnamon bark (*Cinnamomum verum*) reduces triglycerides and increases HDL cholesterol.[56,57]

➢ Lemongrass (*Cymbopogon citratus* or *Cymbopogon flexuosus*) reduces total cholesterol levels when taken orally.[58]

> ➢ Turmeric (*Curcuma longa*) essential oil reduces high cholesterol as effectively as the cholesterol-absorption-limiting drug ezetimibe.[59]
> ➢ Melissa (*Melissa officinalis*) essential oil may reduce triglyceride levels by preventing the creation of fatty acids.[60]

How to use the essential oils
Oral—Take a capsule filled with 5 drops each of cinnamon, lemongrass, and clove morning and evening (adults only).

7

Cough Medicine

Two primary types of medications are used to reduce coughs: suppressants and expectorants. Cough suppressants ease coughs by inhibiting your cough reflex, but they do not help eliminate mucus. Dextromethorphan (DM) is the most common cough suppressant medication. Expectorants help clear the airways by thinning mucus, which makes it easier to expel. Guaifenesin is the most common expectorant used, and the only one approved for use in the United States. DM and guaifenesin may be added to combination medications that utilize both active ingredients. In addition, cough medicines may contain other medicines to relieve associated symptoms, such as decongestants, antihistamines, or painkillers.

Side effects
Dextromethorphan (DM)
- ✓ Blurred vision
- ✓ Drowsiness
- ✓ Dizziness
- ✓ Confusion
- ✓ Difficulty urinating
- ✓ Nausea or severe vomiting
- ✓ Slowed breathing
- ✓ Unusual excitement, nervousness, restlessness, or irritability
- ✓ Shakiness or unsteady movement

   ✓ Constipation
   ✓ Headache
   ✓ Stomach upset
Guaifenesin
   ✓ Diarrhea
   ✓ Dizziness
   ✓ Headache
   ✓ Skin rash
   ✓ Stomachache
   ✓ Headache
   ✓ Hives
   ✓ Nausea or vomiting

Essential oil alternatives

➤ Spike lavender (*Lavandula latifolia*) is considered a useful expectorant.[61]

➤ Tree essential oils (i.e., balsam fir, cypress, and spruce) and those with eucalyptol (eucalyptus, myrtle, lavandin, etc.), also called 1,8-cineole, are commonly used to encourage normal expectoration and respiratory function, including cough reduction.

➤ Eucalyptus (*Eucalyptus globulus*) helps reduce the excess production of mucus caused by both inflammation and respiratory infections.[62,63,64]

➤ Vaporized cinnamon bark (*Cinnamomum verum*) inhibits a number of respiratory pathogens.[65]

➤ Ginger (*Zingiber officinale*) essential oil promotes bronchodilation (dilation of the bronchi in the lungs to improve airflow), which helps improve breathing in people with chronic respiratory diseases.[66] It also reduced the production of pro-inflammatory compounds released during respiratory infections that may restrict airways.[67]

> Inhalation of juniper (*Juniperus communis*) may reduce recurrent upper respiratory tract infections by inhibiting common respiratory pathogens.[68]

> Lemongrass (*Cymbopogon citratus* or *Cymbopogon flexuosus*) inhibits respiratory pathogens.[69]

> A combination of eucalyptus (*Eucalyptus globulus*), myrtle (*Myrtus communis*), sweet orange (*Citrus sinensis*), and lemon (*Citrus limon*) improved mucus clearance from the respiratory system and reduced respiratory inflammation.[70]

> Rosemary (*Rosmarinus officinalis*) rapidly reduces the severity of respiratory tract infections.[71]

How to use the essential oils

Topical—Massage 1 to 2 drops each of eucalyptus, myrtle, cedarwood, and peppermint diluted in carrier oil to the chest and upper back, several times daily; cover chest with a warm, wet rag following application.

Oral—Take a capsule with 3 drops each of oregano, cinnamon, lemongrass, and juniper, 2 to 3 times daily (adults only).

Steam Inhalation—Add 2 drops each of myrtle and eucalyptus, and 1 drop each of juniper and cinnamon to a cup of hot water and inhale for 10 minutes.

8

Cold Medicine

OTC cold medicines are meant to make you more comfortable when you experience a cold, but they do not cure it. They are available as pills, syrups, and nasal sprays. Cold medicines are often categorized as daytime (nondrowsy) and nighttime (help you sleep). These medicines commonly contain a decongestant such as pseudoephedrine and phenylephrine, or an antihistamine to reduce sneezing and runny nose as active ingredients. Nasal sprays contain oxymetazoline and phenylephrine and tend to work much faster than the pills or syrups. If a fever is present, acetaminophen or ibuprofen are usually utilized.

Side effects
- ✓ Elevated heart rate or irregular heart beat
- ✓ Increased blood pressure
- ✓ Drowsiness
- ✓ Thicker mucus secretion
- ✓ Restlessness, nervousness, or anxious feelings
- ✓ Mood swings (easily annoyed or angered)
- ✓ Excessive sweating
- ✓ Dizziness
- ✓ Stomachache or cramps
- ✓ Headache
- ✓ Indigestion
- ✓ Weakness
- ✓ Liver problems

- ✓ Hives, skin rash or eruptions
- ✓ Decreased white blood cell count
- ✓ Hallucinations
- ✓ Nightmares
- ✓ Seizure
- ✓ Nausea or vomiting
- ✓ Difficulty breathing
- ✓ Trembling

Essential oil alternatives
Please refer to the various sections (allergies, cough, fever, and sore throat) for your individual cold symptoms to review the essential oils options for these symptoms.

How to use the essential oils
Please refer to the various sections (allergies, cough, fever, and sore throat) for your individual cold symptoms and how to use the essential oils for these symptoms.

9

Constipation Relievers (Laxatives)

A number of laxatives are available to relieve constipation, each of which works a little differently. The gentlest are bulk-forming laxatives that are also called fiber supplements. When it comes to medications, most commonly used are stimulant laxatives. They should not be used regularly. Stimulant laxatives work by triggering the rhythmic contractions of the bowel called peristalsis. These stimulant laxatives may be administered orally (Dulcolax, Senokot) or rectally (Bisacodyl, Pedia-Lax, Dulcolax). Another drug laxative option is stool softeners (Colace, Surfak) that soften the stool by adding moisture to it, which makes it easier to have a bowel movement without straining.

Side effects
- ✓ Rectal irritation
- ✓ Belching
- ✓ Stomach irritation
- ✓ Cramping
- ✓ Diarrhea
- ✓ Nausea
- ✓ Urine discoloration
- ✓ Interference with nutrient and drug absorption
- ✓ Electrolyte imbalance (which may cause abnormal heart beat, weakness, confusion, and seizures)
- ✓ Dependence to have a bowel movement

Essential oil alternatives
> An abdominal massage with lemon (*Citrus limon*), rosemary (*Rosmarinus officinalis*), and peppermint (*Mentha piperita*) essential oils helped relieve constipation in the elderly.[72]
> Ginger (*Zingiber officinale*) essential oil increases the speed that food travels through the digestive tract, which may relieve constipation.[73]

How to use the essential oils
Topical—Massage 1 drop each of lemon, rosemary, and ginger over the abdomen in a clockwise motion, 1 to 3 times daily, until constipation is relieved.

Oral—Take a capsule with 2 drops each of juniper, ginger, and lemon, 1 to 3 times daily, until constipation is relieved (adults only).

10

Congestion Medications

A variety of different OTC medications are available to relive sinus pressure and pain and nasal congestion. Congestion is often caused by an increased production of mucous in response to inflamed and irritated nasal passages. The increased production of mucous is intended to flush out whatever may be causing the irritation (allergen or pathogen). It is important to keep the nasal passages moist when experiencing congestion because dry nasal passages could increase irritation and the production of mucous. Many of congestion medications combine a pain reliever with a decongestant or antihistamine to attack associated symptoms.

Side effects
- ✓ Coughing
- ✓ Dizziness
- ✓ Drowsiness
- ✓ Fatigue
- ✓ Stomach upset
- ✓ Sore throat
- ✓ Dry mouth
- ✓ Excitability, nervousness, or restlessness
- ✓ Headache
- ✓ Insomnia
- ✓ Nausea or vomiting
- ✓ Weakness

✓ Trembling
✓ Excessive sweating
✓ Irregular heartbeat
✓ Rapid breathing or shortness of breath
✓ Seizure (rare)

Essential oil alternatives

➤ Peppermint (*Mentha piperita*), eucalyptus (*Eucalyptus globulus*), myrtle (*Myrtus communis*), and tree essential oils (balsam fir, cypress, and spruce) are commonly used to open and cleanse the airways and support normal respiratory function.

➤ A combination of eucalyptus (*Eucalyptus globulus*), myrtle (*Myrtus communis*), sweet orange (*Citrus sinensis*), and lemon (*Citrus limon*) improved mucus clearance from the respiratory system and reduced respiratory inflammation.[74]

➤ Topical application of myrtle also reduces inflammation by inhibiting excess leukocyte migration and the proinflammatory molecules TNF-alpha and IL-6, which suggests it will help reduce the nasal inflammation and irritation responsible for the excess mucus production.[75]

➤ Simple nasal irrigation can be an effective way to reduce congestion and nasal symptoms.[76,77]

How to use the essential oils

Topical—Apply 1 to 2 drops of any of the following: eucalyptus, peppermint, or myrtle to the cheeks, nose, chest, and upper back as often as needed.

Steam Inhalation—Place 3 to 4 drops each of eucalyptus and peppermint in a boiling pot of water, and inhale for 10 minutes as often as needed.

Irrigation—Mix together half cup of fine salt or salt flour (not iodized table salt) and 5 drops each of myrtle and rosemary, and 3 drops each of tea tree and lemon essential oils. Store in a sealed glass container. Add ¼ to ½ teaspoon of the mixture to a neti pot and fill with water (distilled, filtered, or boiled and cooled). Irrigate one nostril until the neti pot empties, then repeat the procedure with the other nostril.

11

Depression Medications

Antidepressants are a class of medications used to treat depression by affecting chemicals present in the brain. There are a number of antidepressants available on the market, each targeting depression in a different manner. They are classified according to the neurochemicals they target and affect. Because each type works differently, many people need to try multiple drugs (one at a time) before they find one that works without causing significant side effects.

Atypical antidepressants (Wellbutrin, Remeron, Nefazodone, Oleptro) are unique drugs that don't fit into any other class of antidepressant. They work by modifying levels of chemical messengers (neurotransmitters) in the brain. Depending on the atypical antidepressant, they affect dopamine, serotonin, and norepinephrine levels.

The first class of antidepressant drug developed was monamine oxidase inhibitors (MAOIs). These antidepressants have largely been replaced by other drugs because of their significant side effects. MAOIs work by blocking the monoamine oxidase enzyme from removing the neurotransmitters serotonin, dopamine, and norepinephrine from the brain. This action makes more of these feel-good neurotransmitters available to boost mood and improve brain cell communication.

Selective serotonin reuptake inhibitors, or SSRIs, are the most popular antidepressants prescribed today. They reportedly have fewer and less severe side effects than other depression drugs. They work by blocking the reabsorption of serotonin in the brain. This makes more serotonin available for brain cells to communicate, which in turn boosts mood.

Serotonin and norepinephrine reuptake inhibitors (SNRIs) are used to treat depression, anxiety, and nerve pain. They work by modifying levels of serotonin and norepinephrine in the brain. SNRIs do this by blocking the absorption (reuptake) of both neurotransmitters, which positively influences mood.

Among the earliest drugs developed to treat depression, tricyclic and tetracyclic antidepressants are now generally only prescribed when other safer options have failed to reduce symptoms. They work by blocking the reuptake of serotonin and norepinephrine, but they also affect other chemical messengers, which produces a number of side effects.

Side effects
Atypical antidepressants
   Wellbutrin (bupropion)
- ✓ Headache
- ✓ Weight loss
- ✓ Nausea
- ✓ Loss of appetite
- ✓ Insomnia
- ✓ Fast heartbeat
- ✓ Seizures
- ✓ High blood pressure

Remeron (mirtazapine)
- ✓ Increased appetite
- ✓ Weight gain
- ✓ High cholesterol and triglycerides

Nefazodone
- ✓ Headache
- ✓ Insomnia
- ✓ Weakness
- ✓ Agitation
- ✓ Liver failure
- ✓ Nausea
- ✓ Blurred vision
- ✓ Low blood pressure

Oleptro (trazodone)
- ✓ Headache
- ✓ Blurred vision
- ✓ Extreme fatigue
- ✓ Nausea
- ✓ Diarrhea
- ✓ Irregular heartbeat
- ✓ Muscle aches or pains
- ✓ Sudden drop in blood pressure when standing
- ✓ Sexual dysfunction (persistent, painful erection not associated with sexual arousal)

MAOIs
- ✓ Dry mouth
- ✓ Headache
- ✓ Drowsiness
- ✓ Diarrhea
- ✓ Constipation
- ✓ Nausea
- ✓ Insomnia

- ✓ Dizziness or light-headedness
- ✓ Involuntary muscle movement
- ✓ Low blood pressure
- ✓ Weight gain
- ✓ Muscle aches
- ✓ Difficulty urinating
- ✓ Sexual dysfunction (low desire, difficulty having an orgasm)
- ✓ Tingling sensation in the skin
- ✓ Serious interactions with other medications

SSRIs

- ✓ Nausea
- ✓ Sexual dysfunction (reduced sexual desire, erectile dysfunction, or difficulty reaching orgasm)
- ✓ Nervousness, agitation, or restlessness
- ✓ Drowsiness
- ✓ Insomnia
- ✓ Headache
- ✓ Diarrhea
- ✓ Vomiting
- ✓ Weight gain or loss
- ✓ Dry mouth
- ✓ Serotonin syndrome (dangerously high levels of serotonin)
- ✓ Abnormal bleeding due to interactions with pain relievers and blood pressure medications

SNRIs

- ✓ Dizziness
- ✓ Excessive sweating
- ✓ Dry mouth
- ✓ Nausea
- ✓ Fatigue

- ✓ Difficulty urinating
- ✓ Constipation
- ✓ Insomnia
- ✓ Agitation or anxiety
- ✓ Headache
- ✓ Loss of appetite
- ✓ Sexual problems (reduced desire, difficulty reaching orgasm, erectile dysfunction)
- ✓ Exacerbate liver problems
- ✓ High blood pressure
- ✓ Gastrointestinal bleeding
- ✓ Serotonin syndrome (dangerously high levels of serotonin)

Tricyclic or tetracyclic antidepressants

- ✓ Excessive sweating
- ✓ Constipation
- ✓ Blurred vision
- ✓ Weight gain and increased appetite
- ✓ Dry mouth
- ✓ Difficulty urinating
- ✓ Drowsiness
- ✓ Tremors
- ✓ Low blood pressure when standing
- ✓ Disorientation or confusion
- ✓ Elevated heart rate
- ✓ More frequent seizures among people susceptible to seizures
- ✓ Sexual disorders (decreased sex drive, difficulty reaching orgasm, erectile dysfunction)
- ✓ Serotonin syndrome (dangerously high levels of serotonin)
- ✓ High blood sugar

- ✓ Glaucoma
- ✓ Enlarged prostate
- ✓ Liver disease

Essential oil alternatives

- ➢ Topical application of a 2% dilution (10 drops, three times daily) of orange (*Citrus sinensis*) essential oil reduced depression as well as Prozac.[78] Receiving a regular massage with orange in combination with basil (*Ocimum basilicum*) and geranium (*Pelargonium graveolens*) essential oils also reduced depressive symptoms.[79]
- ➢ Inhaling bergamot (*Citrus bergamia* Risso) essential oil may reduce depressive symptoms.[80]
- ➢ Clary sage (*Salvia sclarea*) reduces depression by influencing dopamine levels.[81]
- ➢ Clove (*Syzygium aromaticum*) essential oil influences hippocampus (an area of the brain associated with depression) function to reduce depression.[82]
- ➢ The inhalation of lemon (*Citrus limon*) influences both dopamine, serotonin, and norepinephrine levels to relieve depression.[83,84]
- ➢ Inhalation of eucalyptus (*Eucalyptus globulus*) significantly increase the release of dopamine.[85]

How to use the essential oils

Topical—Apply a mixture of up to 10 drops of a 2% dilution (about 2 to 3 drops of essential oil per 5 mL of carrier oil) citrus oils (lemon, orange, and bergamot are great options) to a place that won't be exposed to the sun, 1 to 3 times daily.

Inhalation—Place 1 drop each of clove, eucalyptus, and lemon on a tissue and inhale from as needed; refresh the oils on the tissue every 4 to 6 hours.

12

Diarrhea Medications

Emerging evidence now suggests that the huge list of antidiarrheal drugs available on the market are rarely useful and often harmful. Instead, well-informed physicians are now more likely to suggest maintaining hydration and electrolyte balance—possibly combined with a probiotics supplement. However, some diarrheal diseases caused by infections (parasitic or bacterial) will require a prescription. For the purpose of this text, we will focus on two of the most common OTC drugs: loperamide (Imodium) and bismuth subsalicylate (Kaopectate, Pepto-Bismol).

Loperamide works by slowing gastrointestinal motility, allowing more fluid to be absorbed from the intestines. This makes the stools more formed (rather than running and liquid) and reduces diarrhea.

Bismuth subsalicylate combats diarrhea, upset stomach, nausea, and vomiting. It balances fluid movement through the digestive tract, reduces digestive tract inflammation, and prevents the growth of certain pathogens that cause diarrhea.

Side effects
Loperamide
- ✓ Abdominal pain or distension
- ✓ Constipation

- ✓ Dizziness
- ✓ Nausea and vomiting
- ✓ Drowsiness
- ✓ Fatigue
- ✓ Dry mouth
- ✓ Skin rash or itching

Bismuth subsalicylate

- ✓ Constipation
- ✓ Blackened stools or tongue
- ✓ Ringing in the ears or hearing loss
- ✓ Anxiety
- ✓ Headache
- ✓ Confusion
- ✓ Muscle spasms
- ✓ Weakness
- ✓ Reye's syndrome (children under 12)

Essential oil alternatives

- ➢ Peppermint (*Mentha piperita*) slows gastrointestinal motility and reduces intestinal spasms, which may reduce diarrhea.[86,87,88]
- ➢ Myrrh (*Commiphora myrrha*) essential oil inhibits a parasite (fasciola) that is associated with infectious diarrhea.[89]
- ➢ Oregano (*Origanum vulgare*) and nutmeg (*Myristica fragrans*) essential oils inhibit foodborne bacteria associated with diarrhea.[90]
- ➢ Thyme (*Thymus vulgaris*) inhibits a parasite (*G. lamblia*) linked to infectious diarrhea.[91,92]

How to use the essential oils

Oral—Take a capsule with 3 drops each of peppermint and oregano, 1 to 3 times daily, or until diarrhea is relieved (adults only).

Topical—Apply 1 to 3 drops of peppermint and over the abdomen every hour or until diarrhea is relieved.

13

Earache Remedies

Not long ago children with earaches were frequently prescribed antibiotics because earaches are often caused by infections (most commonly bacteria like *Streptococcus pneumoniae, Haemophilus influenzae,* and *Moraxella catarrhalis*). However, the overuse of antibiotics, increase in antibiotic-resistant infections, and the fact antibiotics are not very effective for earaches has lead the American Association of Pediatrics to recommend pain management instead. This leads to use of OTC acetaminophen and ibuprofen to control pain.

Side effects
Please see the section on pain relief medications for the list of possible side effects.

Essential oil alternatives
> - Basil (*Ocimum basilicum*) significantly relieves acute ear infections.[93]
> - Tea tree (*Melaleuca alternifolia*) may reduce inflammation of the ear canal caused by infection.[94]
> - Cinnamon bark (*Cinnamomum verum*), peppermint (*Mentha piperita*), thyme (*Thymus vulgaris*), lemongrass (*Cymbopogon citratus* or *Cymbopogon flexuosus*), and eucalyptus (*Eucalyptus globulus*) all inhibit *S.*

pneumoniae, a common cause of ear infections, and some of them also inhibit *H. influenzae* (another cause of ear infections).[95]

How to use the essential oils
Topical—Apply a mixture of tea tree and basil diluted heavily in carrier oil around the ear (never inside the ear canal) up to 3 times daily. Place 1 drop of basil and tea tree on a cotton ball and place the cotton ball in the ear gently; replace every 30 minutes until symptoms are relieved.

Oral—Take 2 drops each of oregano, lemongrass, cinnamon, and 1 drop each of tea tree, thyme, and eucalyptus in a capsule 3 times daily with a meal (adults only).

14

Fever Reducers

The most common drugs used to reduce fevers are acetaminophen and NSAIDs. In response to infections, your body temperature may temporarily increase to make it less hospitable to harmful organisms that require a narrow temperature range to thrive in. This occurs when concentrations of prostaglandin E(2) (PGE(2)) increase in certain areas of the brain. Elevated PGE(2) levels alter the "firing rate" of neurons that regulate body temperature. Most NSAIDs and acetaminophen work by blocking the action of cyclooxygenase enzymes that subsequently reduce PGE(2) levels.

Side effects
Please see the section on pain relief medications for the list of possible side effects.

Essential oil alternatives
  ➢ Citral, found in abundance in lemongrass (*Cymbopogon citratus* or *Cymbopogon flexuosus*) essential oil, suppresses the COX-2 enzyme.[96]
  ➢ Roman chamomile (*Chamaemelum nobile*) reduces the production of prostaglandins, and suppresses the COX-2 enzyme.[97]
  ➢ Sandalwood (*Santalum album* or *Santalum spicatum*) essential oil reduces the production

of prostaglandins, and suppresses the COX enzymes.[98]

➤ Peppermint (*Mentha piperita*) essential oil stimulates cold receptors on the skin, which causes a sensation of coldness.[99]

➤ Lemon (*Citrus limon*) possesses fever-reducing properties.[100,101]

How to use the essential oils

Topical—Apply trace amounts of peppermint to the tips of the ears, and a drop across the forehead, temples, and back of the neck every 30 minutes until fever reduces (adults). Apply 1 drop of lemon to the spine every 30 minutes until fever reduces (children).

15

First Aid Treatments (Topical Antiseptics)

Topical antiseptics are antimicrobial agents that are applied to the skin to cleanse wounds and prevent infections. These agents kill, inhibit, or reduce a number of microorganisms on the external surfaces of the body that may cause disease. A variety of antiseptics are available, including alcohols, quaternary ammonium compounds, chlorhexidine, chlorine, antibacterial dyes, hypochlorites, diguanides, inorganic iodine, metals, peroxides, and quinolone derivatives.

Side effects
- ✓ Potential damage to healthy skin cells
- ✓ Localized infection at the wound site (usually caused by a contaminated product)
- ✓ Contact dermatitis
- ✓ Chemical burns
- ✓ Hives or rash
- ✓ Itching, redness, or irritation of skin
- ✓ Stinging of skin
- ✓ Skin inflammation
- ✓ Irregular heartbeat
- ✓ Low blood pressure
- ✓ Drowsiness
- ✓ Headache
- ✓ Blurred vision

✓ Central nervous system toxicity
✓ Dizziness
✓ Slowed breathing
✓ Anaphylaxis
✓ Nausea or vomiting

Essential oil alternatives

➤ The majority of essential oils have antiseptic properties to varying degrees.

➤ Tea tree (*Melaleuca alternifolia*) essential oil acts as an antiseptic by activating white blood cells to help fight infections.[102] It also promotes wound healing.[103]

➤ Copaiba (*Copaifera langsdorffii*) essential oil promotes wound healing.[104]

➤ Fennel (*Foeniculum vulgare*) essential oil inhibits the bacterium *Klebsiella pneumoniae*, which is a cause of bloodstream, surgical site, and wound infections.[105]

➤ German chamomile (*Matricaria recutita*) accelerates wound healing.[106]

➤ Research suggests lavender (*Lavandula angustifolia*) may be preferred to Betadine and povidone-iodine for episiotomy wound care.[107,108]

How to use the essential oils

Topical—Mix together 1 tablespoon of witch hazel, 1 teaspoon of aloe vera juice, ¼ teaspoon of vitamin E oil, and 15 drops each of tea tree and copaiba. Shake well and spray on affected area as needed until wound heals.

16

High Blood Pressure Medications

Known as antihypertensives, high blood pressure medications are prescription drugs used to lower high blood pressure (hypertension). There are a variety of classes of high blood pressure medications, including ACE inhibitors, alpha blockers, alpha-2 receptor agonists, angiotensin II receptor blockers, beta blockers, blood vessel dilators (vasodilators), calcium channel blockers, central agonists, diuretics, peripheral adrenergic inhibitors, and renin inhibitors.

ACE inhibitors (angiotensin-converting enzyme inhibitors) decrease blood pressure by blocking the production of angiotensin II. Angiotensin is a peptide hormone that causes the arteries to narrow. Angiotensin-converting enzyme converts angiotensin I to angiotensin II, which causes blood vessel constriction. A reduction in the production of angiotensin II allows the blood vessels to open up and relax, which lowers blood pressure.

Alpha blockers, also called alpha-adrenergic blocking agents, relax the muscle tone of arterial walls, decreasing resistance of blood as it travels through the vessels. They work by blocking the action of norepinephrine, which causes tightening of blood vessels.

Instead of blocking the production of angiotensin II, angiotensin II receptor blockers (ARBs) reduce the cellular response to it. Angiotensin must attach to specific cell receptors to constrict blood vessels. Angiotensin II receptor blockers inhibit angiotensin II from attaching to theses receptors, which maintains open blood vessels and in turn reduces blood pressure.

Beta blockers lower blood pressure by reducing the heart rate, the heart's workload, and the heart's force. They do this by blocking the action of epinephrine (adrenaline). When epinephrine is present in the bloodstream in sufficient quantities, it causes an increase in heart rate, the heart's output of blood, and blood pressure. Some beta blockers also open the blood vessels.

Blood vessel dilators, or vasodilators, decrease blood pressure by relaxing (expanding) the interior walls of blood vessels—especially the arterioles. This action reduces the workload on the heart and decreases blood pressure. ACE inhibitors and nitroglycerine are considered vasodilators.

When calcium enters the smooth muscle cells of the heart and blood vessels, it strengthens the force of heart contractions. Calcium channel blockers prevent calcium from entering these cells, which reduces the force of the heart's contraction, decreases heart rate, opens narrow blood vessels, and reduces blood pressure.

Central agonists (also called central-acting agents or central adrenergic inhibitors) prevent the brain from sending signals to your nervous system that cause the heart rate to increase and the blood vessels to constrict. This action reduces the heart's workload and allows blood to flow more freely through the blood vessels.

Diuretics aid the kidneys in reducing excess sodium (salt) and water through increased urination. The blood vessel walls relax and blood pressure decreases as this unneeded water is removed.

Peripheral adrenergic inhibitors block neuro-transmitters (epinephrine and norepinephrine) from signaling the brain to constrict the blood vessels. These drugs are usually used to treat sever hypertension.

Renin inhibitors block the activity of the enzyme renin, which is involved in blood pressure regulation. Renin, also called angiotensinogenase, is an enzyme secreted by the kidneys that triggers a series of events that converts angiotensinogen to angiotensin I, which is further converted to angiotensin II by ACE. By blocking renin activity, renin inhibitors cause vasodilation and a decrease in blood pressure.

Side effects
ACE inhibitors
- ✓ Headache
- ✓ Diarrhea
- ✓ Rash
- ✓ Chronic dry, hacking cough
- ✓ Drowsiness
- ✓ Loss of sense of taste
- ✓ Kidney damage (rare)
- ✓ Dangers to pregnant mother and baby (low blood pressure, severe kidney failure, excess potassium in the blood, newborn death)

Alpha blockers
- ✓ "First-dose effect" (pronounced low blood pressure and dizziness, which increases the risk of fainting when standing)
- ✓ Headache
- ✓ Pounding heartbeat
- ✓ Nausea
- ✓ Weight gain
- ✓ Weakness

Angiotensin II receptor blockers
- ✓ Dizziness or light-headedness, which may cause fainting when standing from a seated position
- ✓ Diarrhea
- ✓ Vomiting
- ✓ Muscle cramps or weakness
- ✓ Back or leg pain
- ✓ Irregular heartbeat
- ✓ Insomnia
- ✓ Upper respiratory infection
- ✓ Cough
- ✓ Pregnancy complications (injury or death of developing fetus)

Beta blockers
- ✓ Insomnia
- ✓ Fatigue
- ✓ Headache
- ✓ Diarrhea
- ✓ Constipation
- ✓ Upset stomach
- ✓ Depression
- ✓ Cold hands and feet
- ✓ Difficulty breathing

- ✓ Impotence
- ✓ Interactions with diabetic medications

Blood vessel dilators
- ✓ Headaches
- ✓ Swelling around the eyes
- ✓ Joint pain
- ✓ Rapid, pounding, or irregular heartbeat
- ✓ Tingling or numbness in fingers or toes
- ✓ Diarrhea
- ✓ Loss of appetite
- ✓ Upset stomach
- ✓ Flushing of the face or neck
- ✓ Fluid retention or swelling of the ankles
- ✓ Excessive hair growth

Calcium channel blockers
- ✓ Headache
- ✓ Drowsiness
- ✓ Flushing
- ✓ Fluid retention or swollen ankles
- ✓ Dizziness
- ✓ Constipation
- ✓ Rash
- ✓ Nausea
- ✓ Irregular heartbeat

Central agonists
- ✓ Extreme fatigue
- ✓ Impotence
- ✓ Weight gain
- ✓ Headache
- ✓ Psychological problems (depression)
- ✓ Drowsiness
- ✓ Dizziness
- ✓ Constipation

- ✓ Dry mouth
- ✓ Anemia
- ✓ Fever

Diuretics
- ✓ Reduced potassium in the body, which may cause weakness, fatigue, and leg cramps
- ✓ Impotence
- ✓ Upset stomach
- ✓ Nausea
- ✓ Increased skin sensitivity to sunlight
- ✓ Low levels of sodium in the blood
- ✓ Headache
- ✓ Rash
- ✓ Menstrual irregularities
- ✓ Breast enlargement (men)
- ✓ Increased thirst
- ✓ High blood sugar or cholesterol
- ✓ Gout

Peripheral adrenergic inhibitors
- ✓ Heartburn
- ✓ Nasal congestion
- ✓ Diarrhea
- ✓ Dizziness or light-headedness
- ✓ Nightmares
- ✓ Insomnia
- ✓ Depression
- ✓ Impotence

Renin inhibitors
- ✓ Upset stomach or abdominal pain
- ✓ Acid reflux
- ✓ Headache
- ✓ Diarrhea
- ✓ Nasal congestion

- ✓ Hives
- ✓ Dizziness
- ✓ Difficulty breathing
- ✓ Swelling of the face, lips, tongue, or throat

Essential oil alternatives

- ➢ Bergamot (*Citrus bergamia* Risso) essential oil influences calcium levels in cells, reduces endothelial (a thin layer of cells that lines the interior surface of blood vessels) inflammation, and dilates blood vessels, which leads to decreased blood pressure.[109,110,111]
- ➢ Inhaling combinations of essential oils like lavender (*Lavandula angustifolia*), bergamot (*Citrus bergamia* Risso), lemon (*Citrus limon*), marjoram (*Origanum majorana*), neroli (*Citrus aurantium* flowers), and ylang ylang (*Cananga odorata*) reduces blood pressure.[112,113,114]
- ➢ Black pepper (*Piper nigrum*) essential oil inhibits ACE activity.[115]
- ➢ The primary compound found in spearmint (*Mentha spicata*) essential oil, carvone, is a hundred times more potent calcium channel blocker than the drug verapamil.[116]
- ➢ Citronella (*Cymbopogon winterianus*) essential oil, or its major component citronellol, blocks calcium from entering the smooth muscle cells of the heart and blood vessels (calcium channel blocker) and promotes vasodilation.[117,118]

How to use the essential oils

Oral—Take a capsule filled with 5 drops of bergamot and 2 drops each of black pepper, spearmint, and lavender up to twice daily.

Inhalation—Place 1 drop each of bergamot, lemon, lavender, and ylang ylang on a tissue and inhale as needed throughout the day; refresh the oils every 4 to 6 hours.

17

Oral Antiseptics and Rinses

The primary purpose of oral antiseptics and rinses is to disinfect the oral cavity to promote oral hygiene. Disinfecting the oral cavity of microbes can reduce the risk of cavities caused by pathogenic bacteria, reduce plaque, and help maintain gum health. The existence of *Streptococcus mutans* in the oral cavity is strongly associated with cavities; however, this bacterium requires the presence of carbohydrates (sugar) and the enzyme glucosyltransferase (GST) to create acids that attack the teeth. Chlorhexidine gluconate (chlorhexidine for short) is the most common oral antiseptic

Side effects
- ✓ Mouth irritation
- ✓ Teeth staining
- ✓ Dry mouth
- ✓ Unpleasant taste in mouth
- ✓ Altered sense of taste
- ✓ Mouth ulcers or canker sores
- ✓ Coated tongue
- ✓ Parotid gland or salivary gland inflammation

Essential oil alternatives
- ➤ Peppermint is more effective against streptococci and plaque formation than chlorhexidine.[119,120,121]

> ➢ Lemongrass (*Cymbopogon citratus* or *Cymbopogon flexuosus*) essential oil has better antimicrobial properties against clinically significant oral pathogens than chlorhexidine, and a mouthwash containing lemongrass improved gingival index (a measurement of periodontal disease based on severity and location of lesions) better than chlorhexidine.[122,123]

> ➢ Copaiba (*Copaifera langsdorffii*) essential oil inhibits *Streptococcus mutans*, the bacterium considered the primary organism responsible for cavities.[124,125]

> ➢ Lemon (*Citrus limon*) essential oil inhibits GST enzyme activity, which may reduce the risk of cavities.[126]

> ➢ Spearmint (*Mentha spicata*) essential oil prevents *Streptococcus mutans* from sticking together to form tooth plaque.[127]

> ➢ Toothpaste with tea tree (*Melaleuca alternifolia*) essential oil prevents plaque formation and inhibits oral bacteria more effectively than Colgate Total toothpaste.[128] Tea tree mouthwashes also reduce plaque formation and inflammation of the gums.[129]

> ➢ Oregano (*Origanum vulgare*) strongly inhibits *Streptococcus mutans*.[130]

How to use the essential oils

Topical—Add a trace amount of peppermint or lemongrass to your toothpaste before brushing daily. Use a toothpaste that contains any of the above essential oils.

Mouthwash—Mix together 1.5 cups filtered water, 1 tablespoon of aloe vera juice, 1 teaspoon of vegetable glycerin, 1 teaspoon of baking soda, ½ teaspoon of sea salt, 15 drops of peppermint, and 5 drops each of tea tree, spearmint, copaiba, and lemon; shake well and swish with about 2 teaspoons of the mixture for 30 to 60 seconds before spitting.

18

Pain Relief Medications (Acetaminophen and NSAIDs)

Ways to relieve pain are in high demand based on the number of pain killer prescriptions written each year. Astonishingly, enough prescription painkillers were prescribed during 2010 to medicate every American adult every four hours for one month.[131] Prescription pain killers are a major contributor to drug deaths, accounting for over 71 percent of drug deaths—16,235 of the 22,767 deaths that occurred in 2013.[132] There are many different types of OTC and prescription pain killers, including NSAIDs (ibuprofen, naproxen, aspirin, indomethacin, diclofenac, etc.), 5-LOX inhibitors (zileuton, meclofenamate sodium), acetaminophen, and opioids (oxycodone, hydrocodone, meperidine, codeine).

Nonsteroidal anti-inflammatory drugs are the most commonly prescribed medications for inflammatory and painful conditions, such as arthritis. They also reduce fever. NSAIDs are available OTC as ibuprofen and aspirin. They work by preventing enzymes (COX-1, COX-2) from increasing inflammation. The cyclooxygenase-1 (COX-1) enzyme plays a protective role in the body, both defending and playing a role in the production of the stomach lining. The COX-2 enzyme is only present during periods of inflammation. Many NSAIDs reduce the activity of both the COX-1 and COX-2 enzymes, which can produce undesirable effects on the stomach. Some newer drugs target only the COX-2 enzyme (selective COX-2 inhibitors), which is desirable, but they are strongly associated with adverse cardiovascular events.

Another destructive enzyme involved in pain and inflammation is the arachidonate 5-lipoxygenase (5-LOX) enzyme. The 5-LOX enzyme triggers an inflammatory response that is linked to chronic degenerative conditions. Some drugs work by blocking the action of the 5-LOX enzyme, which reduces inflammation and pain.

Acetaminophen is a pain reliever and fever reducer used to relieve mild to moderate pain, such as headache, backache, arthritis, and muscle pain. Taking too much acetaminophen can cause severe liver damage. Unlike NSAIDs, acetaminophen does not reduce inflammation. Instead it works by blocking the creation of chemical messengers called prostaglandins, which are responsible for relaying pain messages and inducing fever. This mechanism of action makes it more likely to relieve pain involving cells of the nervous tissue.

Opioids are highly controlled pain killers available by prescription only because of their extremely addictive nature. They reduce pain intensity by reducing the transmission of pain signals to the brain. Opioids accomplish this by attaching to opioid receptors (found in the brain, spinal cord, gastrointestinal tract, and some other organs) normally occupied by opioids naturally produced in the body (enkephalins, endorphins, dynorphins, and endomorphins). Once attached to the opioid receptors, they send "feel-good" signals to the brain that block pain, slow breathing, and produce a general sense of well-being.

Side effects
NSAIDs
- ✓ Gastrointestinal problems (stomach, esophageal, and small intestine ulcers)
- ✓ Bleeding ulcers or perforation of the stomach or intestines
- ✓ Kidney damage (including kidney failure)
- ✓ Increased risk of heart attack and stroke (especially selective COX-2 inhibitors, but even short-term use of OTC NSAIDs may increase this risk)
- ✓ Reye's syndrome (when administered to children or teenagers with chickenpox or flu-like symptoms)
- ✓ High blood pressure
- ✓ Extreme allergic reactions (especially in those with asthma)
- ✓ Nausea or vomiting
- ✓ Diarrhea
- ✓ Constipation
- ✓ Headache
- ✓ Dizziness
- ✓ Drowsiness
- ✓ Swelling of the arms and legs

5-LOX inhibitors
- ✓ Cough
- ✓ Headache
- ✓ Nausea

- ✓ Upset stomach or abdominal pain
- ✓ Fever
- ✓ Pain or tenderness around the eyes or cheekbones
- ✓ Wheezing or tightness of the chest
- ✓ Difficulty breathing
- ✓ Sore throat
- ✓ Weakness
- ✓ Irregular heartbeat
- ✓ Insomnia
- ✓ Restlessness
- ✓ Flu-like symptoms (rare)
- ✓ Yellow eyes or skin (rare)
- ✓ Suicidal thoughts

Acetaminophen
- ✓ Liver problems (including acute liver failure)
- ✓ Fatal hepatitis (alcoholics)
- ✓ Stomach pain
- ✓ Nausea or vomiting
- ✓ Kidney failure
- ✓ Skin rashes
- ✓ Low blood pressure
- ✓ Headache
- ✓ Insomnia
- ✓ Fatigue
- ✓ Muscle spasms
- ✓ Anxiety
- ✓ Anaphylaxis

Opioids
- ✓ Addiction (physical dependence)
- ✓ Reduced breathing rate
- ✓ Confusion

✓ Overdose (opioids may accumulate over long-term use and cause slowed breathing, seizures, and decreased heartbeat)
✓ Sexual dysfunction (impotence, difficulty achieving orgasm)
✓ Drowsiness
✓ Restlessness
✓ Muscle or joint pain
✓ Dizziness
✓ Itching
✓ Nausea or vomiting
✓ Constipation
✓ Unconsciousness or coma

Essential oil alternatives:

➢ Basil (*Ocimum basilicum* linalool CT) essential oil influences pain pathways in the central nervous system and reduces prostaglandins to relieve pain.[133,134]

➢ Eucalyptus (*Eucalyptus globulus*) binds to opioid receptors (central analgesic) and blocks the production of substances that cause pain (peripheral analgesic).[135]

➢ Bergamot (*Citrus bergamia* Risso) essential oil influences the nervous system to reduce pain— even pain caused by something that would not normally cause pain.[136]

➢ Cassia (*Cinnamomum cassia*) essential oil blocks COX-2 and prostaglandins while simultaneously increasing the release of anti-inflammatory compounds (IL-10, transforming growth factor-beta).[137]

➢ Lemongrass (*Cymbopogon citratus* or *Cymbopogon flexuosus*) essential oil inhibits COX-2 and the release of proinflammatory cytokines (IL-1beta and IL-6).[138,139] It reduces pain and inflammation as well as the NSAID lysine acetylsalicylic (Aspirin DL-lysine).[140] It possesses both central and peripheral analgesic properties that make it useful for nerve pain.[141]

➢ Myrtle (*Myrtus communis*) relieves pain and inflammation as well as the prescription NSAID indomethacin.[142]

➢ Sandalwood (*Santalum album*) essential oil inhibits cytokines, chemokines, prostaglandins, and COX enzymes about as well as ibuprofen.[143] It also strongly inhibits the 5-LOX enzyme.[144]

➢ Cedarwood (*Cedrus atlantica*) essential oil moderately inhibits the 5-LOX enzyme; whereas, Himalayan cedarwood (*Cedrus deodora*) strongly inhibits the 5-LOX enzyme.[145] Remarkably, inhalation of cedarwood (*Cedrus atlantica*) activates opioid pathways that reduce pain.[146]

➢ Copaiba (*Copaifera langsdorffii*) essential oil strongly inhibits the 5-LOX enzyme and reduces both peripheral and central pain.[147,148]

➢ Lemon (*Citrus limon*), orange (*Citrus sinensis*), and tangerine (*Citrus reticulata*) essential oils strongly inhibit the 5-LOX enzyme.[149]

➢ Rosemary (*Rosmarinus officinalis*) essential oil interacts with adrenergic receptors to relieve pain.[150]

➤ A combination of marjoram (*Origanum majorana*), black pepper (*Piper nigrum*), lavender (*Lavandula angustifolia*), and peppermint (*Mentha piperita*) reduces neck pain and increases range of motion in people with a history of neck pain.[151]

➤ Massaging the knee with ginger (*Zingiber officinale)* and orange (*Citrus sinensis*) essential oil reduces pain and increase knee function.[152]

➤ Application of peppermint (*Mentha piperita*) essential oil and ethanol to the forehead and temples relieved headaches.[153]

How to use the essential oils
Oral—Take 5 drops of copaiba, and 3 drops each of lemongrass, bergamot, and myrtle in a capsule up to 3 times daily.

Topical—Rub 1 to 2 drops (sufficient to cover the area) each of ginger, black pepper, basil, and peppermint essential oil in about 1 teaspoon of carrier oil to the affected area up to 3 times daily.

19

Sleep Remedies

Sometimes an underlying medical disorder is the cause of insomnia, but if no medical or sleep disorder is present, a hypnotic sleeping pill may be prescribed. There are two primary types of sleeping pills: benzodiazepines (flurazepam, triazolam, temazepam, diazepam, alprazolam, and lorazepam) and , also called benzodiazepine receptor agonists or "Z-drugs" (zolpidem, eszopiclone, and zaleplon). Benzodiazepines depress the central nervous system by enhancing the activity of the neurotransmitter GABA (gamma aminobutyric acid). Nonbenzodiazepines also affect GABA but are more targeted in their approach, affecting only certain parts of the GABA receptor. A newer sleep aid called Rozerem targets melatonin receptors instead. Antidepressants may also be prescribed as a sleep aid because of their influence on serotonin and norepinephrine levels, which can cause a sedating effect. Diphenhydramine is an antihistamine that is also used as an OTC sleeping pill because it has sedating effects.

Side effects
- ✓ Addiction (physical dependence)
- ✓ Drowsiness
- ✓ Memory loss
- ✓ Unsteadiness and falls

✓ Hung-over feeling
✓ Dizziness
✓ Heartburn
✓ Light-headedness
✓ Headache
✓ Muscle aches
✓ Constipation
✓ Dry mouth or throat
✓ Gastrointestinal upset
✓ Diarrhea
✓ Unusual dreams
✓ Nausea
✓ Prolonged drowsiness
✓ Severe allergic reactions
✓ Abnormal sleep behaviors (eating, driving, or making phone calls while sleeping)
✓ Mental performance problems or trouble concentration

Essential oil alternatives

➢ Inhalation of lavender (*Lavandula angustifolia*) essential oil may improve sleep quality among individuals with disturbed sleep patterns.[154,155] It has also been shown to increase GABA activity.[156]

➢ Vetiver stimulates GABA activity and depresses the central nervous system to promote relaxation and sleep.[157,158]

➢ Cedarwood (*Cedrus deodora*) essential oil significantly enhances GABA levels in the brain.[159]

How to use the essential oils

Inhalation—Diffuse a combination of 2 drops each of lavender, cedarwood, and vetiver 30 minutes prior to sleeping. Place 1 drop each of lavender, cedarwood, and vetiver on an aroma stone next to the bed while sleeping.

Topical—Massage 1 drop each of lavender, cedarwood, and vetiver to the feet at least 15 minutes prior to going to bed.

Oral—Take 2 drops each of lavender, cedarwood, and vetiver in a capsule 30 minutes before going to bed.

20

Sore Throat Remedies

The majority of sore throats are caused by viral infections like those responsible for colds and flus. They can also be caused by bacterial infections, such as strep throat—which is caused by *Streptococcus pyogenes* or group A streptococcus. In addition, allergies, dry air, air pollution, strain from yelling, GERD, or tumors can cause a sore throat. Viral infections may be treated with combination OTC medicines like those designed to reduce cold and flu symptoms. Antibiotics are the treatment of choice for strep throat infections that cause a sore throat.

Side effects (depending on the antibiotic)
- ✓ Alteration of the gut microbiome
- ✓ Allergic hypersensitivity reactions
- ✓ Rash
- ✓ Headache
- ✓ Dizziness
- ✓ Diarrhea
- ✓ Changes in the sense of taste, or a metallic taste in the mouth
- ✓ Lethargy
- ✓ Colitis
- ✓ Jaundice
- ✓ Abdominal pain
- ✓ Nausea or vomiting
- ✓ Fever
- ✓ Vaginal candidiasis

- ✓ Kidney or liver toxicity
- ✓ Elevated white blood cells
- ✓ Flushing
- ✓ High blood pressure

Essential oil alternatives

- ➢ Peppermint (*Mentha piperita*), thyme (*Thymus vulgaris*), cinnamon (*Cinnamomum verum*), and lemongrass (*Cymbopogon citratus* or *Cymbopogon flexuosus*) essential oils all inhibit *Streptococcus pyogenes* (a bacterium that causes strep throat and tonsillitis).[160]
- ➢ Eucalyptus (*Eucalyptus globulus*) inhibits *Streptococcus pyogenes* (a bacterium that causes strep throat and tonsillitis).[161,162]
- ➢ Tea tree (*Melaleuca* alternifolia) essential oil protects against *Streptococcus A* infections.[163]
- ➢ Marjoram (*Origanum majorana*) significantly inhibits *Streptococcus A*.[164]

How to use the essential oils

If the sore throat is caused by a viral infection (cold, flu, mononucleosis, croup, etc.), please see the recipes for each condition outlined in *Evidence-Based Essential Oil Therapy*.

For strep throat:

Oral—Take a capsule filled with 3 drops each of lemongrass, marjoram, cinnamon, and peppermint, and 1 drop each of eucalyptus and tea tree, 3 to 4 times daily. Gargle with a 1 drop each of lemongrass, peppermint, and marjoram in 1 teaspoon of honey and a glass of warm water every couple hours.

REFERENCES

[1] Thomson Reuters. 2015 CMR Pharmaceutical R&D Factbook. Global pharma sales to reach $1.3 trillion. Accessed January 26, 2016 from http://thomsonreuters.com/en/articles/2015/global-pharma-sales-reach-above-1-trillion.html.

[2] Axxess Pharma Inc. Accessed January 26, 2016 from http://www.financialnewsmedia.com/profiles/axxe.html.

[3] f 17:1-58.

[4] OpenSecrets.org. Pharm/Health Prod, 2015. Accessed January 26, 2015 from http://www.opensecrets.org/lobby/indusclient_lobs.php?id=h04&year=2015.

[5] OpenSecrets.org. Top Industries. Accessed January 26, 2016 from https://www.opensecrets.org/lobby/top.php?indexType=i.

[6] World Health Organization. Pharmaceutical Industry. Accessed January 26, 2016 from http://www.who.int/trade/glossary/story073/en/.

[7] The Commonwealth Fund. Mirror, Mirror on the Wall, 2014 Update: How the U.S. Health Care System Compares Internationally. Accessed January 26, 2016 from http://www.commonwealthfund.org/publications/fund-reports/2014/jun/mirror-mirror.

[8] U.S. Food and Drug Administration. FDA Drug Safety Communication: FDA strengthens warning that non-aspirin nonsteroidal anti-inflammatory drugs (NSAIDs) can cause heart attacks or strokes. http://www.fda.gov/Drugs/DrugSafety/ucm451800.htm.

[9] Fontana RJ. Acute Liver Failure including Acetaminophen Overdose. Med Clin North Am. Author manuscript; available in PMC 2009 Jul 1.

[10] Singh S, Loke YK, Furberg CD. Thiazolidinediones and Heart Failure: A teleo-analysis. Diabetes Care. 2007 Aug;30(8):2148-2153.

[11] Lewis JD, Ferrara A, Peng T, et al. Risk of bladder cancer among diabetic patients treated with pioglitazone: interim report of a longitudinal cohort study. Diabetes Care. 2011;34:916-22.

[12] Tomljenovic L, Shaw CA. Too fast or not too fast: the FDA's approval of Merck's HPV vaccine Gardasil. J Law Med Ethics. 2012 Fall;40(3):673-81.

[13] U.S. Centers for Disease Control and Prevention. Vaccine Safety: Frequently asked questions about HPV vaccine safety.

Accessed February 2, 2016 from
http://www.cdc.gov/vaccinesafety/vaccines/hpv/hpv-safety-faqs.html.

[14] National Vaccine Safety Information Center. Med Alerts: Found 218 cases where Vaccine is HPV4 or HPV9 and Patient Died and Submission Date on/before '2015-12-31'. Accessed February 2, 2016 from
http://www.medalerts.org/vaersdb/findfield.php?TABLE=ON&GROUP1=AGE&GROUP2=VCT&GRAPH=ON&GROUP6=AGE&EVENTS=ON&VAX[]=HPV4&VAX[]=HPV9&DIED=Yes&WhichAge=range&LOWAGE=&HIGHAGE=&SUB_YEAR_HIGH=2015&SUB_MONT.

[15] Brinth L, Theibel AC, Pors K, et al. Suspected side effects to the quadrivalent human papilloma vaccine. Dan Med J. 2015 Apr;62(4):A5064.

[16] Brinth LS, Pors K, Theibel AC, et al. Orthostatic intolerance and postural tachycardia syndrome as suspected adverse effects of vaccination against human papilloma virus. Vaccine. 2015 May 21;33(22):2602-5.

[17] Moro PL, Zheteyeva Y, Lewis P, et al. Safety of quadrivalent human papillomavirus vaccine (Gardasil) in pregnancy: adverse events among non-manufacturer reports in the Vaccine Adverse Event Reporting System, 2006-2013. Vaccine. 2015 Jan 15;33(4):519-22.

[18] Harris T, Williams DM, Fediurek J, et al. Adverse events following immunization in Ontario's female school-based HPV program. Vaccine. 2014 Feb 19;32(9):1061-6.

[19] Gatto M, Agmon-Levin N, Soriano A, et al. Human papillomavirus vaccine and systemic lupus erythematosus. Clin Rheumatol. 2013 Sep;32(9):1301-7.

[20] Lexchin J. New Drugs and Safety: What Happened to New Active Substances Approved in Canada Between 1995 and 2010? Arch Intern Med. 2012;172(21):1680-1681.

[21] Kalemba D, Kunicka A. Antibacterial and Antifungal Properties of Essential Oils. Curr Med Chem. 2003 May;10(10):813-29.

[22] Baratta MT, Dorman HJD, Deans SG, et al. Antimicrobial and antioxidant properties of some commercial essential oils. Flav Farg J. 1998 July-Aug;13(4):235-44.

[23] Aydin S, Özturk Y, Beis R, et al. Investigation of Origanum onites, Sideritis congesta and Satureja cuneifolia Essential Oils for Analgesic Activity. Phytother Res. 1996 Jun;10(4):342-44.

[24] Cosentino S, Tuberoso CIG, Pisano B, et al. In-vitro antimicrobial activity and chemical composition of Sardinian Thymus essential oils. Letters in Applied Microbiology. 1999 Aug;29:130–135.

[25] Santos FA, Rao VSN. Antiinflammatory and Antinociceptive Effects of 1,8-Cineole a Terpenoid Oxide Present in many Plant Essential Oils. Phytother Res. 2000;14:240-44.

[26] Johnson S. Evidence-Based Essential Oil Therapy: The Ultimate Guide to the Therapeutic and Clinical Application of Essential Oils. 2015. Orem, Utah: Scott A Johnson Professional Writing Services, LLC.

[27] Johnson S, Plant J. Synergy, It's an Essential Oil Thing: Revealing the Science of Essential Oil Synergy with Cells, Genes, and Human Health. 2015. Orem, Utah: Scott A Johnson Professional Writing Services, LLC.

[28] Aisenberg W, Pluznick J. Localization of a novel renal olfactory receptor to glomeruli. FASEB J. 2013;27:lb856.

[29] Pluznick JL, Zou DJ, Zhang X, et al. Functional expression of the olfactory signaling system in the kidney. PNAS. Proc Natl Acad Sci U S A. 2009 Feb 10;106(6):2059-64.

[30] Spehr M, Gisselmann G, Poplawski A, et al. Identification of a testicular odorant receptor mediating human sperm chemotaxis. Science. 2003 Mar 28;299(5615):2054-8.

[31] American College of Preventive Medicine. Over-the-counter medications: Use in general and special populations, therapeutic errors, misuse, storage and disposal. Accessed January 27, 2016 from http://www.acpm.org/?OTCMeds_ClinRef

[32] Shinde UA, Kulkarni KR, Phadke AS, et al. Mast cell stabilizing and lipoxygenase inhibitory activity of Cedrus deodara (Roxb.) Loud. Wood oil. Indian J Exp Biol. 1999 Mar;37(30):258-61.

[33] Mitoshi M, Kuriyama I, Nakayama H, et al. Effects of essential oils from herbal plants and citrus fruits on DNA polymerase, cancer cell growth inhibitory, anti-allergenic, and antioxidant activities. J Agric Food Chem. 2012 nov;60(145):11343-50.

[34] Kim HM, Cho SH. Lavender oil inhibits immediate-type allergic reaction in mice and rats. J Pharm Pharmacol. 1999 Feb;51(2):221-26.

[35] Mitoshi M, Kuriyama I, Nakayama H, et al. Suppression of allergic and inflammatory responses by essential oils derived

from herbal plants and citrus fruits. Int J Mol Med. 2014 Jun;33(6):1643-51.

[36] Koh KJ, Pearce AL, Marshman G, et al. Tea tree reduces histamine-induced skin inflammation. Br J Dermatol. 2002 Dec;147(6):1212-17.

[37] Ferrara L, Naviglio D, Armone Caruso A. Cytological aspects on the effects of a nasal spray consisting of standardized extract of citrus lemon and essential oils in allergic rhinopathy. ISRN Pharm. 2012;2012:404606.

[38] Juergens JR. Anti-inflammatory properties of the monoterpene 1,8-cineole: Current evidence for co-medication in inflammatory airway diseases. Drug Res (Stuttg).2014 Dec;64(12):638-46.

[39] Hammad H, Chieppa M, Perros F, et al. House dust mite allergen induces asthma via Toll-like receptor 4 triggering of airway structural cells. Nat Med.2009 Apr;15(4):410-16.

[40] Lu XQ, Tang FD, Wang Y, et al. Effect of Eucalyptus globulus oil on lipopolysaccharide-induced chronic bronchitis and mucin hypersecretion in rats. Zhongguo Zhong Yao ZA Zhi. 2004 Feb;29(2):168-71.

[41] Boschi F, Nicolato E, Benati D, et al. Drug targeting of airway surface liquid: a pharmacological MRI approach. Biomed Pharmacother. 2008 Jul-Aug;62(6):410-19.

[42] Yamahara J, Huang QR, Li YH, et al. Gastrointestinal motility enhancing effect of ginger and its active constituents. Chem Pharm Bull (Tokyo). 1990 Feb;38(2):430-31.

[43] Kamiya T, Adachi H, Joh T. [Relationship between gastric motility and the pathophysiology of GERD]. Nihon Rinsho. 2007 May;65(5):836-9.

[44] Weseler A, Geiss HK, Saller R, et al. A novel colorimetric broth microdilution method to determine the minimum inhibitory concentration (MIC) of antibiotics and essential oils absent Helicobacter pylori. Pharmazie. 2005 Jul;60(7):498-502.

[45] Deriu A, Branca G, Molicotti P, et al. In vitro activity of essential oil of Myrtus communis L. against Helicobacter pylori. Int J Antimicrob Agents. 2007 Dec;30(6):562-63.

[46] Imai H, Osawa K, Yasuda H, et al. Inhibition by the essential oils of peppermint and spearmint of the growth of pathogenic bacteria. Microbios. 2001;106 Suppl 1;31-39.

[47] Jamal A, Javed K, Aslam M, et al. Gastroprotective effect of cardamom, Elettaria cardamomum Maton. fruits in rats. J Ethnopharmacol. 2006 Jan;103(2):149-53.

[48] Santin JR, Lemos M, Kelin-Júnior LC, et al. Gastroprotective activity of essential oils of the Syzygium aromaticum and its major component eugenol in different animal models. Naunyn-Schmiedeberg's Arch Pharmacol. 2011 Feb;383(2):149-58.

[49] Paiva LA, Rao VS, Garmosa NV, et al. Gastroprotective effect of Copaifera langsdorffii ole-resin on experimental gastric ulcer models in rats. J Ethnopharmacol. 1998 Aug;62(1):73-78.

[50] Al-Howiriny T, Alsheikh A, Alqasoumi S, et al. Protective effect of Origanum majorana L. 'Marjoram" on various models of gastric mucosal injury in rats. Am J Chin Med. 2009;37(3):531-45.

[51] Wilkins J Jr. Method for treating gastrointestinal disorder.US patent (642045). 2002.

[52] Willette RC, Barrow L, Doster R, et al. Purified d-limonene: an effective agent for the relief of occasional symptoms of heartburn. Proprietary study. WRC Laboratories, Inc. Galveston, TX.

[53] Grundy SM, Mok HY, Zech L, Berman M. Influence of nicotinic acid on metabolism of cholesterol and triglycerides in man. J Lipid Res. 1981 Jan;22(1):24-36.

[54] Schmid F, Christeller S, Rehm W. Studies on the state of vitamins B1, B2 and B6 in Down's syndrome. Fortschr Med. 1975;93(25):1170-1172.

[55] Nikolaevskiĭ VV, Kononova NS, Pertsovskiĭ AI, et al. Effect of essential oils on the course of experimental atherosclerosis. Patol Fiziol Eksp Ter. 1990 Sep-Oct;(5):52-53.

[56] Ping H, Zhang G, Ren G. Antidiabetic effects of cinnamon oil in diabetic KK-Aγ mice. Food Chem Toxicol. 2010 Aug-Sep;48(8-9):2344-49.

[57] Kim SH, Hyun SH, Choung SY. Anti-diabetic effect of cinnamon extract on blood glucose in db/db mice. J Ethnopharmacol. 2006 Mar;104(1-2):119-123.

[58] Costa CA, Bidinotto LT, Takahira RK, et al. Cholesterol reduction and lack of genotoxic or toxic effects in mice after repeated 21-day oral intake of lemongrass (Cymbopogon citratus) essential oil. Food Chem Toxicol. 2011 Sep;49(9):2268-72.

[59] Singh V, Jain M, Misra A, et al. Curcuma oil ameliorates hyperlipidaemia and associated deleterious effects in golden Syrian hamsters. Br. J Nutr. 2013 Aug 28;110(3):437-46.

[60] Jun HJ, Lee JH, Jia Y, et al. Melissa officinalis essential oil reduces plasma triglycerides in human apolipoprotein E2

transgenic mice by inhibiting sterol regulatory element-binding protein-1c-dependent fatty acid synthesis. J Nutr. 2012 Mar;142(3):432-40.

[61] Charron JM. Use of Lavandula latifolia as an expectorant. J Altern Complement Med. 1997 Fall;3(3):211.

[62] Juergens JR. Anti-inflammatory properties of the monoterpene 1,8-cineole: Current evidence for co-medication in inflammatory airway diseases. Drug Res (Stuttg).2014 Dec;64(12):638-46.

[63] Hammad H, Chieppa M, Perros F, et al. House dust mite allergen induces asthmas via Toll-like receptor 4 triggering of airway structural cells. Nat Med.2009 Apr;15(4):410-16.

[64] Lu XQ, Tang FD, Wang Y, et al. Effect of Eucalyptus globulus oil on lipopolysaccharide-induced chronic bronchitis and mucin hypersecretion in rats. Zhongguo Zhong Yao ZA Zhi. 2004 Feb;29(2):168-71.

[65] Inouye S, Takizawa T, Yamaguchi H. Antibacterial activity of essential oils and their major constituents against respiratory tract pathogens by gaseous contact. J Antimicrob Chemother. 2001 May;47(5):565-73.

[66] Mangprayool T, Kupittayanant S, Chudapongse N. Participation of citral in the bronchodilatory effect of ginger oil and possible mechanism of action. Fitoterapia. 2013 Sep;89:68-73.

[67] Podlogar JA, Verspohl EJ. Antiinflammatory effects of ginger and some of its components in human bronchial epithelial (BEAS-2B) cells. Phytother Res. 2012 Mar;26(3):333-36.

[68] Camporese A. In vitro activity of Eucalyptus smithii and Juniperus communis oils against bacterial biofilms and efficacy perspectives of complementary inhalation therapy in chronic and recurrent upper respiratory tract infections. Infez Med. 2013 Jun;21(2):117-24.

[69] Inouye S, Takizawa T, Yamaguchi H. Antibacterial activity of essential oils and their major constituents against respiratory tract pathogens by gaseous contact. J Antimicrob Chemother. 2001 May;47(5):565-73.

[70] Lai Y, Dilidaer D, Chen B, et al. In vitro studies of a distillate of rectified essential oils on sinonasal components of mucociliary clearance. Am J Rhino Allergy. 2014 May-Jun;28(3):244-48.

[71] Ben-Arye E, Dudai N, Eini A, et al. Treatment of upper respiratory tract infections in primary care: A randomized study using aromatic herbs. Evid-Based Complement Altern Med. 2011;2011:690346.

[72] Kim MA, Sakong JK, Kim EJ, et al. Effect of aromatherapy massage for the relief of constipation in the elderly. Taehan Kanho Hakhoe Chi. 2005 Feb;35(1):56-64.

[73] Yamahara J, Huang QR, Li YH, et al. Gastrointestinal motility enhancing effect of ginger and its active constituents. Chem Pharm Bull (Tokyo). 1990 Feb;38(2):430-31.

[74] Lai Y, Dilidaer D, Chen B, et al. In vitro studies of a distillate of rectified essential oils on sinonasal components of mucociliary clearance. Am J Rhino Allergy. 2014 May-Jun;28(3):244-48.

[75] Maxia A, Frau MA, Falconieri D, et al. Essential oil of Myrtus communis inhibits inflammation in rats by reducing serum IL-6 and TNF-alpha. Nat Prod Commun. 2011 Oct;6(10):1545-48.

[76] Tomooka LT, Murphy C, Davidson TM. Clinical study and literature review of nasal irrigation. Laryngoscope. 2000;110(7):1189-93.

[77] Hermelingmeier KE, Weber RK, Hellmich M, et al. Nasal irrigation as an adjunctive treatment in allergic rhinitis: A systematic review and meta-analysis. Am J Rhinology Allergy. 2012 Sep-Oct;26(5):e119-e125.

[78] Sargolzaee MR, Fayyazi Bordbar MR, Shakiba M, et al. The comparison of the efficacy of Citrus Fragrance and Fluoxetine in the treatment of major depressive disorder. J of Gonabad University of Med Sci and Health Sci. 2004;10(3):43-48.

[79] Okamoto A, Kuriyama H, Watanabe S, et al. The effect of aromatherapy massage on mild depression: A pilot study. Psych Clin Neurosci. 2005 Jun;59(3):363.

[80] Lemon K. An assessment of treating depression and anxiety with aromatherapy. Int J Aromatherapy. 2004 Jul;14(2):63-69.

[81] Seol GH, Shim HS, Kim PJ, et al. Antidepressant-like activity effect of Salvia sclarea is explained by modulation of dopamine activities in rats. J Ethnopharmacol. 2010 Jul 6;130(1):187-90.

[82] Seol GH, Shim HS, Kim PJ, et al. Antidepressant-like activity effect of Salvia sclarea is explained by modulation of dopamine activities in rats. J Ethnopharmacol. 2010 Jul 6;130(1):187-90.

[83] Komiya M, Takeuchi T, Harada E. Lemon oil vapor causes an antistress effect via modulating the 5-HT and DA activities in mice. Behav Brain Res. 2006 Sep;172(2):240-49.

[84] Kiecolt-Glaser JK, Graham JE, Malarkey WB, et al. Olfactory influences on mood and autonomic, endocrine, and immune function. Psychoneuroendocrinology. 2008 Apr;33(3):328-39.

[85] Kako H, Fukumoto S, Kobayashi Y, et al. Effects of direct exposure of green odour components on dopamine release from rat brain striatal slices and PC12 cells. Brain Res Bull. 2008 Mar;75(5):706-12.

[86] Asao T, Mochiki E, Suzuki H, et al. An easy method for the intraluminal administration of peppermint oil before colonoscopy and its effectiveness in reducing colon spasms. Gastrointest Endosc. 2001 Feb;53(2):172-77.

[87] Liu JH, Chen GH, Yeh HZ, et al. Enteric-coated peppermint-oil capsules in the treatment of irritable bowel syndrome: a prospective, randomized trial. J Gastroenterol. 1997;32:765-68.

[88] Goerg KJ, Spilker T. Effect of peppermint oil and caraway oil on gastrointestinal motility in healthy volunteers: a pharmacodynamic study using simultaneous determination of gastric and gall-bladder emptying and orocaecal transit time. Ailment Pharmacol Ther. 2003 Feb;17(3):445-51.

[89] Massoud A, El Sisi S, Salama O, et al. Preliminary study of therapeutic efficacy of a new fasciolicidal drug derived from Commiphora molmol (myrrh). Am J Trop Med Hyg. 2001 Aug;65(2):96-99.

[90] Firouzi R, Shekarforoush SS, Nazer AH, et al. Effects of essential oils of oregano and nutmeg on growth and survival of Yersinia enterocolitica and Listeria monocytogenes in barbecued chicken. J Food Prot. 2007 Nov;70(11):2626-30.

[91] Machado M, Dinis AM, Salquiero L, et al. Anti-giardia activity of phenolic-rich essential oils: effects of Thymbra capitata, Origanum virens, Thymus zygis subsp. Sylvestris, and Lippia graveolens on trophozoites growth, viability, adherence, and ultrastructure. Parasitol Res. 2010 Apr;106(5):1205-15.

[92] Machado M, Sousa Mdo C, Salgueiro L, et al. Effects of essential oils on the growth of Giardia lamblia trophozoites. Nat Prod Commun. 2010 Jan;5(1):137-41.

[93] Kristinsson KG, Magnusdottir AB, Petersen H, et al. Effective treatment of experimental acute otitis media by application of volatile fluids into the ear canal. J Infect Dis. 2005 Jun 1;191(11):1876-80.

[94] Farnan TB, McCallum J, Awa A, et al. Tea tree oil: in vitro efficacy in otitis externa. J Laryngol Otol. 2005 Mar;119(3):198-201.

[95] Inouye S, Takizawa T, Yamaguchi H. Antibacterial activity of essential oils and their major constituents against respiratory tract pathogens by gaseous contact. J Antimicrob Chemother. 2001 May;47(5):565-73.

[96] Katsukawa M, Nakata R, Takizawa Y, et al. Citral, a component of lemongrass oil, activates PPARa and y and suppressed COX-2 expression. Biochem Biophys Acta. 2010 Nov;1801(110:1214-20.

[97] Srivastava JK, Pandey M, Gupta S. Chamomile, a novel and selective CoX-2 inhibitor with anti-inflammatory activity. Life Sci. 209 Nov;85(19-20):663-69.

[98] Sharma M, Levenson C, Bell RH, et al. Suppression of liposaccharide-stimulated cytokine/chemokine production in skin cells by sandalwood oils. Phyther Res. 2014 Jun;28(6):925-32.

[99] No author listed. Peppermint: Drugdex Drug Evaluations, Micromedex Inc. Healthcare Series, 1999.

[100] Arteche García, A., 1998. Fitoterapia: Vademécum de Prescripción. Masson, Barcelona.

[101] Arias BA, Ramón-Laca L. Pharmacological properties of citrus and their ancient and medieval uses in the Mediterranean region. J Ethnopharm. 2005;97:89-95.

[102] Budhiraja SS, Cullum ME, Sioutis SS, et al. Biological activity of Melaleuca alternifolia (Tea Tree) oil component, terpinen-4-ol, in human myelocytic cell line HL-60. J Manipulative Ther. 1999 Sep;22(7):447-53.

[103] Pazyar N, Yaghoobi R, Bagherani N, et al. A review of applications of tea tree oil in dermatology. Int J Dermatol. 2013 Jul;52(7):784-90.

[104] Paiva LA, de Alencar Cunha KM, Santos FA, et al. Investigation of the wound healing activity of ole-resin from Copaifera langsdorffii in rats. Phytother Res. 2002 Dec;16(8):737-39.

[105] Tripathi P, Tripathi R, Patel RK, et al. Investigation of antimutagenic potential of Foeniculum vulgare essential oil on cyclophosphamide induced genotoxicity and oxidative stress in mice. Drug Chem Toxicol.2013 Jan;36(1):35-41.

[106] Domingues Martins M, Martins Marques M, Kalil Bussadori S, et al. Comparative analysis between Chamomilla recutita and corticosteroids on wound healing. An in vitro and in vivo study. Phytother Res. 2009;23:274-78.

[107] Sheikhan F, Jahdi F, Khoei EM, et al. Episiotomy pain relief: Use of lavender essence in primiparous Iranian women. Complement Ther Clin Pract. 2012 Feb;18(1):66-70.

[108] Vakilian K, Atarha M, Bekhradi R, et al. Healing advantages of lavender essential oil during episiotomy recovery: a clinical trial. Complement Ther Clin Pract. 2011 Feb;17(1):50-53.

[109] Kang P, Han SH, Moon HK, et al. Citrus bergamia Risso elevates intracellular CA (2+) in human vascular endothelial cells due to release of Ca (2+) from primary intracellular stores. Evid Based Complement Altern Med. 2013;2013:759615.

[110] Kang P, Suh SH, Min SS, et al. The essential oil of Citrus bergamia Risso induces vasorelaxation of the mouse aorta by activating K(+) channels and inhibiting Ca(2+) influx. J Pharm Pharmacol. 2013 May;65(5):745-49.

[111] You JH, Kang P, Min SS, et al. Bergamot essential oil differentially modulates intracellular Ca2+ levels in vascular endothelial and smooth muscle cells: a new finding seen with fura-2. J Cardiovasc Pharmacol. 2013 Apr;61(4):324-28.

[112] Hwang JH. The effects of the inhalation method using essential oils on blood pressure and stress responses of clients with essential hypertension. Taehan Kanho Hakhoe Chi. 2006 Dec;36(7):1123-34.

[113] Hwang JH. The effects of the inhalation method using essential oils on blood pressure and stress responses of clients with essential hypertension. Taehan Kanho Hakhoe Chi. 2006 Dec;36(7):1123-34.

[114] Kim IH, Kim C, Seong K, et al. Essential oil inhalation on blood pressure and salivary cortisol levels in prehypertensive and hypertensive subjects. Evid Based Complement Alternat Med. 2012;2012:984203.

[115] Oboh G, Ademosun AO, Odubanjo OV, et al. Antioxidative properties and inhibition of key enzymes relevant to type-2 diabetes and hypertension by essential oils from black pepper. Adv Pharmacol Sci. 2013;2013:926047.

[116] Souza FV, da Rocha MB, de Souza DP, et al. (-)-Carvone: antispasmodic effect and mode of action. Fitoterapia. 2013 Mar;85:20-24.

[117] de Menezes IA, Moreira IJ, de Paula JW, et al. Cardiovascular effects induced by Cymbopogon winterianus essential oil in rats: involvement of calcium channels and vagal pathway. J Pharm Pharmacol. 2010 Feb;62(2):215-21.

[118] Dzumayev KK, Tsibulskaya IA, Zenkevich IG, et al. Essential oils of Salvia sclarea L. produced from plants grown in Southern Uzbekistan. J Essential Oil res. 1995;7(6):597-604.

[119] Rasooli I, Shayegh S, Taghizadeh M, et al. Phytotherapeutic prevention of dental biofilm formation. Phytother Res. 2008 Sep;22(9):1162-67.

[120] Shayegh S, Rasooli I, Taghizadeh M, et al. Phytotherapeutic inhibition of supragingival dental plaque. Nat Prod Res. 2008 Mar 20;22(5):428-39.
[121] Shapiro S, Meier A, Guggenheim B. The antimicrobial activity of essential oils and essential oil components towards oral bacteria. Oral Microbiol Immunol. 1994 Aug;9(4):202-08.
[122] Karbach J, Ebenezer S, Warnke PH, et al. Antimicrobial effect of Australian antibacterial essential oils as alternative to common antiseptic solutions against clinically relevant oral pathogens. Clin Lab. 2015;61(1-2):61-68.
[123] Dany SS, Mohanty P, Tangade P, et al. Efficacy of 0.25% lemongrass oil mouthwash: A three arm prospective parallel clinical study. J Clin Diagn Res. 2015 Oct;9(10):ZC13-17.
[124] Souza AB, Martins CH, Souza MG, et al. Antimicrobial activity of terpenoids from Copaifera langsdorffii Desf. against cariogenic bacteria. Phytother Res. 2011 Feb;25(2):215-20.
[125] Pieri FA, Mussi MCM, Fiorini JA, et al. Bacteriostatic effect of copaiba oil (Copaifera officinalis) against Streptococcus mutans. Braz Dent J. 2012;23(1):0103-6440.
[126] Shi YF, Zhang XY, Han H, et al. Effect of lemon essential oil on caries factors of Streptococcus sobrinus. Ahonqhua Kou Qiang Yi Xue Za Zhi. 2012 Dec;47(12):739-42.
[127] Rasooli I, Shayegh S, Astaneh S. The effect of Mentha spicata and Eucalyptus camaldulensis essential oil on dental biofilm. Int J Dent Hyg. 2009 Aug;7(3):196-203.
[128] Santamaria M Jr, Petermann KD, Vedovello SA, et al. Antimicrobial effect of Melaleuca alternifolia dental gel in orthodontic patients. Am J Orthod Dentofacial Orthop. 2014 Feb;145(2):198-202.
[129] Saxer UP, Stauble A, Szabo SH, et al. Effect of mouthwashing with tea tree oil on plaque and inflammation. Schweiz Monatsschr Zahnmed. 2003;113(9):985-96.
[130] 1626 Miller AB, Cates RG, Lawrence M, et al. The antimicrobial and antifungal activity of essential oils extracted from Guatemalan medicinal plants. Pharm Biol. 2015 Apr;53(4):548-54.
[131] United Nations Office on Drugs and Crime. World Drug Report 2011. Accessed January 28, 2016 from http://www.unodc.org/documents/data-and-analysis/WDR2011/World_Drug_Report_2011_ebook.pdf
[132] U.S. Centers for Disease Control and Prevention. Prescription Drug Overdose Data. Deaths from prescription opioid overdose.

Accessed January 28, 2016 from
http://www.cdc.gov/drugoverdose/data/overdose.html.
[133] Nascimento SS, Araujo AA, Brito RG, et al. Cyclodextrin-complexed Ocimum basilicum leaves essential oil increases Fos protein expression in the central nervous system and produce an antihyperalgesic effect in animal models for fibromyalgia. Int J Mol Sci. 2014 Dec 29;16(1):547-63.
[134] Venâncio AM, Onfre AS, Lira AF, et al. Chemical composition, acute toxicity, and antinociceptive activity of the essential oil of plant breeding cultivar of basil (Ocimum basilicum L.). Planta Med. 2011 May;77(8):825-29.
[135] Silva J, Abebe W, Sousa SM, et al. Analgesic and anti-inflammatory effects of essential oils of eucalyptus. J Ethnopharmacol. 2003 Dec;89(2-3):277-83.
[136] Sakurada T, Kuwahata H, Katsuyama S, et al. Intraplantar injection of bergamot essential oil into mouse hindpaw: effects on capsaicin-induced nociceptive behaviors. Int Rev Neurobiol. 2009;85:237-48.
[137] Pannee C, Chandhanee I, Wacharee L. Anti-inflammatory effects of essential oils from the leaves of Cinnamomum cassia and cinnamaldehyde on lipopolysaccharide-stimulated J774A.1 cells. J Adv Pharm Technol Res. 2014 Oct;5(4):164-70.
[138] Sforcin JM, Amaral JT, Fernandes A Jr, et al. Lemongrass effects on IL-1beta and IL-6 production by macrophages. Nat Prod Res. 2009;23(12):1151-59.
[139] Katsukawa M, Nakata R, Takizawa Y, et al. Citral, a component of lemongrass oil, activates PPARa and y and suppressed COX-2 expression. Biochem Biophys Acta. 2010 Nov;1801(110:1214-20.
[140] Gbenou JD, Ahounou JF, Akakpo HB, et al. Phytochemical composition of Cymbopogon citratus and Eucalyptus citriodora essential oils and their anti-inflammatory and analgesic properties on Wistar rats. Mol Biol Rep. 2013 Feb;40(2):1127-34.
[141] Viana GS, Vale TG, Pinho RS, et al. Antinociceptive effect of the essential oil from Cymbopogon citratus in mice. J Ethnopharmacol. 2000 Jun;70(3):323-27.
[142] Nassar MI, Aboutabl el-SA, Ahmed RF, et al. Secondary metabolites and bioactives of Myrtus communis. Pharmacognosy Res. 2010 Nov;2(6):325-29.
[143] Sharma M, Levenson C, Bell RH, et al. Suppression of liposaccharide-stimulated cytokine/chemokine production in

skin cells by sandalwood oils. Phyther Res. 2014 Jun;28(6):925-32.

[144] Baylac S, Racine P. Inhibition of 5-lipoxygenase by essential oils and other natural fragrance extracts. Int J Aromatherapy. 2003;13(2-3):138-42.

[145] Baylac S, Racine P. Inhibition of 5-lipoxygenase by essential oils and other natural fragrance extracts. Int J Aromatherapy. 2003;13(2-3):138-42.

[146] Martins DF, Emer AA, Paula Batisti A, et al. Inhalation of Cedrus atlantica essential oil alleviates pain behavior through activation of descending pain modulation pathways in a mouse model of postoperative pain. J Ethnopharmacol. 2015 Sep 3. [Epub ahead of print]

[147] Baylac S, Racine P. Inhibition of 5-lipoxygenase by essential oils and other natural fragrance extracts. Int J Aromatherapy. 2003;13(2-3):138-42.

[148] Gomes NM, Rezende CM, Fontes SP, et al. Antinociceptive activity of Amazonian copaiba oils. J Ethnopharmacol. 2007 Feb;19(3):486-92.

[149] Baylac S, Racine P. Inhibition of 5-lipoxygenase by essential oils and other natural fragrance extracts. Int J Aromatherapy. 2003;13(2-3):138-42.

[150] Sagorchev P, Lukanov J, Beer AM. Investigations into the specific effects of rosemary oil at the receptor level. Phytomedicine. 2010 Jul;17(8-9):693-97.

[151] Ou MC, Lee YF, Li CC, et al. The effectiveness of essential oils for patients with neck pain: a randomized controlled study. J Altern Complement Med. 2014 Oct;20(10):771-79.

[152] Yip YB, Tam AC. An experimental study on the effectiveness of massage with aromatic ginger and orange essential oil for moderate-to-severe knee pain among the elderly in Hong Kong. Complement Ther Med. 2008 Jun;16(3):131-38.

[153] Göbel H, Schmidt G, Dworschak M, et al. Essential plant oils and headache mechanism. Phytomedicine. 1995 Oct;2(2):93-12.

[154] Lytle J, Mwatha C, Davis KK. Effect of lavender aromatherapy on vital signs and perceived quality of sleep in the intermediate care unit: a pilot study. Am J Crit Care. 2014 Jan;23(1):24-29.

[155] Lis-Balchin M. Studies on the mode of action of the essential oil of lavender (Lavandula angustifolia P. Miller). Phytother Res. 1999 Sep;13(6):540-42.

[156] Bradley BF, Starkey NJ, et al. Anxiolytic effects of Lavandula angustifolia odour on the Mongolian gerbil elevated plus maze. J Ethnopharmacol. 2007;111:517–25.

[157] Maignana Kumar R, Rukmani A, Saradha S, et al. Evaluation of antiepileptic activity of vetiveria zizanioides oil in mice. Int J Pharm Sci Rev Res. 2014 Mar-Apr;25(2):248-51.

[158] de Sousaa DP, Nóbregab FF, de Morais LC, et al. Evaluation of the Anticonvulsant Activity of Terpinen-4-ol. Z Naturforsch C. 2009 Jan-Feb;64(1-2):1-5.

[159] Viswanatha GL, Nandakumar K, Shylaja H, et al. Anxiolytic and Anticonvulsant activity of alcoholic extract of heart wood of Cedrus deodara Roxb. in rodents. J Pharm Res Health Care. 2009;1:217-239.

[160] Inouye S, Yamaguchi H, Takizawa T. Screening of the antibacterial effects of a variety of essential oils on respiratory tract pathogens, using a modified dilution assay method. J Infect Chemother. 201 Dec;7(4):251-54.

[161] Cermelli C, Fabio A, Fabio G, et al. Effect of eucalyptus essential oil on respiratory bacteria and viruses. Curr Microbiol. 2008 Jan;56(1):89-92.

[162] Salari MH, Amine G, Shirazi MH, et al. Antibacterial effects of Eucalyptus globulus leaf extract on pathogenic bacteria isolated from specimens of patients with respiratory tract disorders. Clin Microbiol Infect. 2006 Feb;12(2):194-96.

[163] Tsao N, Kuo CF, Lei HY, et al. Inhibition of group A streptococcal infection by Melaleuca alternifolia (tea tree) oil concentrate in the murine model. J Appl Microbiol. 2010 Mar;108(3):936-44.

[164] 1312 Hamida-Ben Ezzeddine NB, Abdelkefi MM, Aissa RB, et al. Antibacterial screening of Origanum majorana L. oil from Tunisia. J Essent Oil Res. 2001;13(4):295-97.

ABOUT THE AUTHOR

Dr. Scott A. Johnson is the bestselling author of nine books and more than 300 articles featured in online and print publications. He is the creator and founder of the Integrative Essential Oils Essential Oil Certification Program, and the originator of the Waterfall Technique™. He has a doctorate in naturopathy, is a board-certified alternative medical practitioner (AMP), Certified Elite Essential Oil Specialist (CEEOS), Certified Clinical Master Aromatherapist (CCMA), and Certified Professional Coach (CPC). His evidence-based approach to natural healing and experience conducting medical research make him one of the world's leading experts on the therapeutic application of essential oils. Dr. Johnson pioneered evidence-based essential oil therapy, which combines the art of ancient healing with modern science to maximize the benefits of essential oils. One of his research focuses is the safety of essential oils, and he has published internationally on the subject. He is an acclaimed international speaker and has delivered keynote presentations across North America, Europe, and Asia. Dr. Johnson draws on his wealth of experience and diverse educational background as he travels the globe to share the secrets of natural healing with those who seek greater wellness.

Connect with Dr. Johnson

Twitter: @DocScottJohnson

Facebook: /AuthorScottAJohnson

Website: authorscott.com

Discover more books by Dr. Scott A. Johnson

Evidence-Based Essential Oil Therapy: The Ultimate Guide to the Therapeutic and Clinical Application of Essential Oils

Surviving When Modern Medicine Fails: A definitive guide to essential oils that could save your life during a crisis

Synergy, It's an Essential Oil Thing: Revealing the Science of Essential Oil Synergy with Cells, Genes, and Human Health

The Doctor's Guide to Surviving when Modern Medicine Fails: The Ultimate Natural Medicine Guide to Preventing Disease and Living Longer

Beating ADHD Naturally

TransformWise: Your Complete Guide to a Wise Body Transformation

Beating Ankylosing Spondylitis Naturally

The Word of Wisdom: Discovering the LDS Code of Health

Jeremy's Christmas Journey (Fictional book and musical CD)

Get certified in the safe and effective use of essential oils with Dr. Johnson's comprehensive and evidence-based program:

The Integrative Essential Oils Certification Program

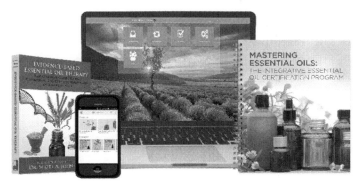

ieocertified.com

INDEX

A

B

C

INDEX

D

E

F

INDEX

INDEX

M

MAOIs, 59
marketing, 11, 12, 17
markets, pharmaceutical, 10
mast cells, 35, 36, 37
medical-grade, 25-26
Merck, 17
microbial testing, 27

N

niacin, 43, 44
Nitropress, 15
nonbenzodiazepines, 97
norepinephrine, 59, 60, 64, 77, 79, 97
NSAIDs, 89-95

O

optical rotation, 26
oral administration, 24-25
organoleptic, 27

P

painkillers, 47, 89
peripheral adrenergic inhibitors, 77, 79, 82
PGE(2), 73
physicians, 3, 10, 11, 43, 67
potency, 32
profit, 14, 15, 18, 19, 25

INDEX

INDEX